WHY CHILDHOOD ILLNESS MATTERS
Lyndsey Hookway

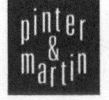

Why Childhood Illness Matters (Pinter & Martin Why It Matters 27)
First published by Pinter & Martin Ltd 2023

©2023 Lyndsey Hookway

Lyndsey Hookway has asserted her moral right to be identified as the author of this work in accordance with the Copyright, Designs and Patents Act of 1988.

All rights reserved

ISBN 978-1-78066-665-5

Also available as an ebook

Pinter & Martin Why It Matters ISSN 2056-8657

Series editor: Susan Last
Index: Helen Bilton
Cover Design: Blok Graphic, London
British Library Cataloguing-in-Publication Data

A catalogue record for this book is available from the British Library.

This book is sold subject to the condition that it shall not, by way of trade and otherwise, be lent, resold, hired out, or otherwise circulated without the publisher's prior consent in any form or binding or cover other than that in which it is published and without a similar condition being imposed on the subsequent purchaser.

Set in Minion

Printed and bound in the UK by Clays

This book has been printed on paper that is sourced and harvested from sustainable forests and is FSC accredited.

Pinter & Martin Ltd
Unit 803 Omega Works
4 Roach Road
London E3 2PH

pinterandmartin.com

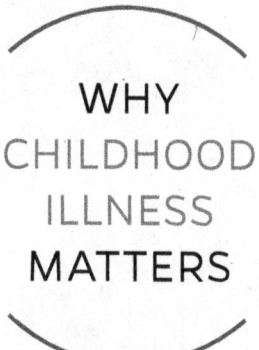

WHY CHILDHOOD ILLNESS MATTERS

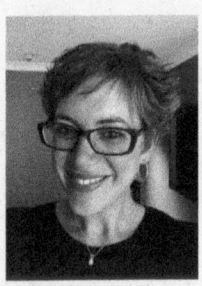

About the author

Lyndsey Hookway is a paediatric nurse, health visitor, IBCLC, responsive sleep influencer, and researcher. The mother of a childhood sepsis and cancer survivor, she often talks about the impact of chronic childhood illness on families, and seeks to support other families living through serious illness. Her research focuses on the needs and challenges of medically complex breastfed infants and children, as well as their families, and the health professionals caring for them. She is the author of *Holistic Sleep Coaching* (2018), *Let's talk about your new family's sleep* (2020), *Still Awake* (2021) and *Breastfeeding the Brave* (2022).

Contents

Introduction	7
1 How illness makes parents feel	13
2 Types of illness	29
3 On the ward	45
4 Family-centred care	64
5 Treatments and procedures	79
6 Caring for children with complex illnesses, conditions, and disabilities	97
7 Childhood illness and sleep	118
8 The impact of illness on families, and how to support them	133
Conclusion	153
Resources	155
Acknowledgements	158
References	159
Index	170

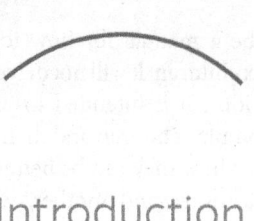

Introduction

The number of children who are admitted to hospital has increased over the last 10 years, with 2.9 million children admitted per year in 2016. More than half a million of these admissions were for a child under the age of four (Keeble and Kossarova, 2017). 39% of these children attended the emergency department before being admitted. That doesn't even include all those children who were admitted via a non-emergency route. These are vast numbers. Childhood illness matters because it is likely that you or someone you know has been affected by it.

More and more families are living with a chronic childhood illness or condition and, happily, many of these children will spend much of their time at home, or in the community. This means that professionals who are not paediatric clinicians may increasingly encounter these fabulous families and wonder what their needs are and how to support them given their ongoing condition.

This book is not about how parents and children use hospital and healthcare services, or the state of the NHS. It's not intended to be a manual for how to clinically manage medically complex children. It will not delve into the intricacies of specific conditions. It is intended to provide insight into what medically complex children and their families face, what their needs are, and how they can be better supported.

As a paediatric nurse and mother, what I'm interested in are the human experiences of healthcare. Thousands of parents watch their child becoming unwell at home. They debate who to call for advice, and whether to go to the doctor. They might decide to go to A&E or call an ambulance. They sit. They endure children's TV on a loop in the waiting area. They wonder how many infectious children have mouthed the toys before their child did. They wait. They worry. They try desperately to understand NHS-language. What did the doctor mean when they said that? Why is that nurse looking anxious? When's my child's turn? Is my child really unwell? Did I pack enough nappies? Did I feed the cat before I left? Did I turn the oven off before the paramedics loaded us into the ambulance? Will I have to call in sick for work tomorrow? Will my child be okay?

Thousands of families per year have their lives turned upside down for an afternoon, 24 hours, a week, several months, or even more. Half a million families per year navigate a hospital admission, endure separation and disruption, and sleep a night or more away from home. Medical complexity throws up a variety of practical, emotional, relational, psychological and clinical problems – and the more people who know how to support these families in a wider sense, the better.

Every experience of caring for a sick child, whether in a parenting or professional capacity, is different. Of course, we know which acute illnesses are most common. We know that viral infections, bronchiolitis, respiratory infections, gastrointestinal infections and tonsillitis are likely to be the

Introduction

reason a child ends up in hospital. We know that asthma, diabetes and epilepsy are the most common chronic illnesses of childhood. We know which medicines and supportive treatments will probably help and which guidelines to follow. We know on average how long those children will spend as in-patients. We know children's care is getting more complex and what the possible complications are (Kanthimathinathan, 2020). But that's about all we know when it really comes down to it. Working with children is a test of humility; of acknowledging that while a disease process may follow a predictable path, exactly how that plays out is variable.

When I first trained as a children's nurse in 2001, one of the first core messages I received was that children only make sense in the context of the family and environment in which they are being raised. This means that the way a child responds is likely to be a product not only of their illness, but also their genetics, their parenting, their innate personality, and their family. That's what makes them fascinating – in my opinion! In child health, you never just care for a child. You care for a child *and* someone special. You are probably caring for a child, someone special, and some other people back home too. In fact, you are caring for a child, someone special, their family at home, and all the details of the life back home that went on hold as soon as that child became unwell. It's never *just* a child.

As a parent, caring for a child means directing your attention in several different directions. Looking after them, having fun with them, meeting their needs, doing your best, knowing you're not perfect but getting on with it anyway. Negotiating how your child's life dovetails with your own, your other children, their schooling, the finances that make it all possible. Caring for a sick child is more complicated, because a parent's instinct will be to ignore all those spinning plates and focus wholly on their child. But real life doesn't make that easy. The bills don't go away. The other children need love and care too. A parent's job won't get done by itself. The house won't clean itself and you can bet your life there's no fairy to do the laundry either. The spinning plates crash around these families, adding to the general chaos and anxiety.

While childhood illness is common, it is also profoundly abnormal, and requires understanding and adaptions by the child, family, community and medical team. Half a million families every year know this all too well. Half a million families worried, panicked and stressed. But also – half a million families somehow coped, overcame and showed courage and strength.

One of those families was mine. I know firsthand what it's like to sit in A&E. To wait for the triage nurse. To hear them fast bleep the doctor. To watch the numbers on the screen go up, go down, flash, alarm and bleep. To see people come running. To have my unresponsive child removed from my arms so that lifesaving care can be given. To receive a diagnosis nobody wants to hear. As well as being a paediatric and public health nurse, I'm also the mother of a childhood sepsis and cancer survivor. I have been on the paediatric ward *in* and *out* of uniform and I can see both sides.

This book is written for and about families of sick children so that those providing support understand a little of their world. I may not know about an individual journey, but I know a little of the trials, dramas, despair and anxiety along the way. I also know that there is beauty lurking deep within the ugliest of situations. There are profoundly humbling, funny and poignant moments that deserve to be spoken about. There is immense strength and resilience to be found in ordinary humans experiencing extraordinary challenges. Finally, these children deserve to be honoured, validated, and respected for the huge amounts of bravery and steadfastness in adversity that they show every day. I am in awe of them.

Who is this book for?

Children with medical complexity live among us. There are hidden disabilities and chronic conditions that families are so good at coping with you could be forgiven for not knowing the drama that they quietly deal with. Other times illness is obvious and so are the challenges. Either way, whether you are the parent of a sick or medically complex child, or you are supporting families of sick children, this book aims to support *you*.

You may be a doula, booked to support a family who have an antenatal diagnosis of a major congenital anomaly. You might be the preschool teacher of a child with a chronic illness. You could be the IBCLC supporting an infant who is recovering from a life-threatening condition. Perhaps you're a sleep coach supporting a child who has a disability. You may also be a parent of a sick child. If you are, I'm so glad you're here. Please feel free to take what you need from this book, and leave what you don't. I'm also acutely conscious that there may be stories or topics in this book which feel close to your reality. Just skip anything you don't need to read right now, and make sure you hand this book to someone who can support you.

More and more children are living and thriving with illnesses, conditions and disability. Many of these families, happily, are integrating with mainstream school and accessing services in the community. But some parents reach out for additional help or get creative and look for support outside the standard care provided by hospital services and settings. This is wonderful and means that a rich variety of expertise and skills can be tapped into. Services everywhere are stretched, and it makes sense to utilise skills that are within the community. The only problem is that many people in the community offering support may not have any clinical paediatric training. They may not understand the pressures of hospitals or the hundreds of directions that paediatric clinicians are pulled in. After all, it is hard to understand a system you have never been part of. There may be misunderstandings or misinterpretations. Professionals in the community may only hear a version of events given by an exhausted and stressed parent. This book aims to demystify paediatric healthcare experiences and thus give a balanced view of what goes on: a kind of paediatric interpreter if you will.

Understanding how childhood illness affects children and families is crucial because illness cannot be neatly compartmentalised, allowing you to focus only on your job. The tentacles of medical complexity reach into almost every other area, and understanding this is essential to provide compassionate, joined-up care, separate illness from wellness, and advocate for families who may need additional input. Illness affects children and families across multiple different domains, and of course, everyone is unique, which means that the same illness will manifest differently for two children. But briefly, childhood illness affects a child's quality of life, affects both their and their family's psychological wellbeing, has impacts on peers, indirectly affects education, opportunities and play, directly and indirectly affects the relationship they have with their parents and siblings, and may also have both short and long-term effects. Sometimes these effects can be minimised, and at other times they need to be understood and managed, but realising the wider-reaching impacts is the first step. My hope is that all who read this will have a greater sense of awareness of the lived experiences of families facing childhood illness.

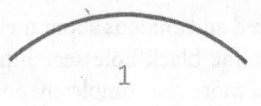

1
How illness makes parents feel

You might legitimately wonder why I'm starting a book about childhood illness with how the illness affects the parent. This is not to diminish the impact that illness has on children (I'll get to that!), but rather it is an acknowledgement that parents are usually the first interface between professionals and sick children. For most parents, childhood illness can bring about some intense emotions. Anger. Grief. Confusion. Shock. Disappointment. Whether they knew their child's condition before they were born, or they have been handed a diagnosis at some point later on, they will undoubtedly feel a bewildering array of feelings. They may feel afraid that it is somehow their fault (it almost certainly isn't). They may wonder 'why *my* child?', only to then quickly feel guilty because they wouldn't wish this on anyone. They may wish they could take their child's illness upon themselves, to spare them the treatment or problems they will face. They may be angry at those around them with healthy children, despising those who complain about seemingly trivial problems when they perceive that they have a bigger mountain to climb. They may feel bewildered and anxious about their child's prognosis, or fall into an online black hole searching for answers. All these feelings and more are completely normal. They are not odd, and they are also not alone.

> 'As a parent I felt like I'd lost complete control of my life. Something I wish I had known was just how much statistics can vary. Because so many studies for rare diagnoses are based on really small population sizes there is a lot of room for the unique circumstance of your child to play a big role and create a unique outcome.' Brittney Piper

In many ways, living with childhood illness is a 'new' problem. We are benefitting from decades of research into improving the survival and quality of life of children with illness. As little as 30–50 years ago, many of the conditions that now have high cure rates were fatal. We simply don't, therefore, have a whole lot of evidence about what the reality of living with long-term conditions is like for families (Compas et al, 2012). We are in uncharted territory; moving (happily) from a position of simply being grateful for survival, to learning about how to *thrive*.

Many families need to *learn* how to thrive through illness. Because it deviates from the typical course of childhood, thriving through adversity requires adaptations. It may initially cause a 'rabbit-in-headlights' response as parents realise that aspects of family life they had planned may now need altering.

Childhood illness is many things, but I think above everything else it is a thief. It (tries to) steal joy, fun, family time, togetherness, carefree days, normality, socialising, school days, hijinks and laughter. However, if families can lean in, develop coping mechanisms, and accept some adaptations, they can minimise some of the impacts. I don't mean you

How illness makes parents feel

can stop the course of the illness. I don't mean that it will be easy. But over the years I've learnt that leaning in can develop character, resilience and grace that people didn't know they were capable of. Families will discover that the friends and family who matter are the ones who show up. They will learn that bravery isn't the absence of fear, but the quiet, steadfast perseverance despite it. They will learn that as a parent, they can't always make everything okay, but they can make things better simply by being there.

When we were told we would 'kick cancer's butt', I think people meant that we would overcome it and achieve remission. In truth, kicking cancer's butt for us meant the maintenance of eternal optimism and a child not stunted or stained despite cancer. That, for me, is the real success. My hope for families is that they can hold on to hope, learn to lean on others, not be afraid of vulnerability and raw emotion, and fiercely protect the character of the child they are fighting for.

'My daughter has an unknown issue which results in her being unable to eat and having global developmental delay. I find it really hard to be around other children her age or younger, as I see where she "should" be and the delays become more apparent, so I isolate myself from friends and hide them on social media, so I don't have to see how their children are. I struggle with accepting the "wait and see" plan from the NHS, meaning I have had to become a ferocious advocate and fight for my daughter.

So how do I feel as a parent? Isolated. Angry. Blamed. Guilty. Exhausted. Despondent. Invisible. Terrified. Abandoned.

But for all the negatives, I still have my wonderful, beautiful, determined daughter who brings such joy to my life. I just wish I felt supported and cared for so

> *I could enjoy being her mother rather than being an unpaid carer and advocate as well.'* <u>Gemma Hamilton</u>

I wish children didn't become unwell – I really do. But given that this is unrealistic, the next best option is that families are supported to become pragmatic about their experience. Yes, they may be dented and bruised. But they may also become more human versions of themselves. More humble. More grateful. More compassionate. Working with and for families of sick children is an extraordinary privilege.

How childhood illness affects *you*

It would be remiss of me to fail to acknowledge that the carers, supporters and cheerleaders of children and families may be directly or vicariously affected by the challenges and trauma of illness. Firstly, it is not easy to witness another human going through hardship, especially if you work in a role that demands high levels of empathy. Secondly, none of us are immune to childhood illness – perhaps you are yourself a childhood illness survivor, or your children have had their (un)fair share of illness or medical complexity. Indeed, many people are drawn to work with certain populations *because* of their own personal experiences.

If you relate to this, you'll need to take care of yourself for several reasons.

1. You may find it triggering to look after a family if their situation reminds you strongly of a personal experience. You may be a parent as well, or you might have personal experience of childhood illness – perhaps you, a family member or a friend. This may mean that you need to say no to working with some families to protect yourself from unexpected difficult or heavy feelings. Trauma and triggers

can affect us when we least expect it.
2. If you work with lots of families who are dealing with childhood illness you may find, particularly if you are a highly empathic person, that your grief and overwhelm bucket becomes full. Working with and for families who are enduring hardship and difficulty is emotionally exhausting and we all need time to relax and switch off or we risk burnout. Of course, taking a break is not always as easy or even possible for the amazing families that you support, but that's a wholly separate issue.
3. Finally, the other risk of working with many families with childhood illness is over-identification. If we are exposed disproportionately to a particular condition, we can begin to 'see' it all over the place. It can be risky from a scope of practice point of view because experience and exposure does not necessarily equate to expertise. It is also risky to take on families with a particular condition if it is something you have personal experience of, because we can sometimes fall into the trap of recommending things that worked personally. Objectivity is important, so stepping away, referring on, and broadening your client base may be a safer strategy.

The grief and disappointment of illness

It is important to recognise the uniqueness of a family's story, whatever the child's illness. Some children have a congenital condition that they will live with for the rest of their life. Other children may have weeks, months or years of challenges. A child's illness may be acute or chronic. They may spend time in intensive care, or become more familiar with the children's outpatient department waiting room than they would have liked. They may have surgery to overcome, or daily medications. A child's condition may present itself in a dramatic way, with ambulances, running and loud beeping machines. Or it may be calm, delivered over a conversation and a cup of hospital-grade tea.

None of these different presentations of illness or complexity is 'better' than another, although there is some evidence that longer lasting conditions are very different to those of a shorter duration. Chronic conditions (those lasting more than three months and requiring multiple hospitalisations or medical treatments) have been found to be more stressful. However, what is interesting is that the severity of a child's illness does not seem to be a factor in predicting parental stress (Franck et al, 2015). Rather, it seems to be the disruption to family life that many parents find challenging.

Some parents feel guilty for finding their child's condition difficult. You may hear phrases along the lines of 'we're lucky she doesn't have X – that would be worse', or 'we don't have it as bad as some'. This tendency to minimise is something I have seen many times in stoic and stalwart parents, but they are not in competition with anyone else. Their child's illness and challenges are unique to them. The impact on their family is unique and significant. They don't have to justify their situation to anyone.

This minimisation may come from a slight lean towards institutionalisation. Multiple hospital admissions expose parents to many other different families' experiences of illness, and they may feel guilty for finding their child's diabetes difficult when the family opposite is dealing with a major road traffic accident. The medical teams around the child may also unwittingly contribute to the 'putting a brave face on it' attitude because their exposure to childhood illness is significant and they have more perspective and objectivity. At times this may appear as a blasé or unemotional pragmatism about illness, which can seem cold or unconcerned. However, the reality is that paediatric health professionals *do* care about

How illness makes parents feel

children as well – they simply cannot fall apart every time a child is sick.

The paediatric staff may be reassuring and optimistic, but a parent's experience is what they say it is. It's okay (and normal) to be sad, scared, and angry at times. Ultimately, while all of this might be an everyday occurrence to a healthcare professional, it is often a unique experience for a parent. Unwittingly, some parents can fall into the trap of minimising illness as well. When we were first transferred to a major cancer specialist centre, it felt like everyone was playing cancer 'top trumps'. Conversations in the parents' coffee lounge always got around to 'so, what's your kid got then?' and everyone knew that the pecking order was being established. Who's got the worst/most unusual diagnosis? Who do we tiptoe around? The truth is that there are no 'good' cancers. No 'good' diagnoses of congenital heart disease. No 'good' diagnoses of diabetes. No 'good' diagnoses of pneumonia, or sepsis, sickle cell disease, major multiple allergies, or [insert the child's medical condition here]. Families are not in a pecking order, and their story is their own. What all parents have in common is that it is not what they planned.

At the heart of this is that almost all parents have aspirations for their child. These aspirations may vary based on our own experiences of childhood, our culture or community. Sometimes we might imagine or dream about our child's future. Some parents might say that they value learning and academic success. Others might place a higher value on kindness and likeability. Often, though, when all those higher-level desires are stripped away, we simply desire our children to be happy and healthy. A diagnosis of either acute or chronic illness attacks this primal desire for health at the core. Part of the grief that parents feel is this sense of coming to terms with the difference between the dream and the reality.

Numbness

Children are part of a family. There is a large body of evidence that acknowledges the impact of childhood illness on parents, as well as children. After all, children are a product of the family and environment in which they are raised. Some parents feel like they can't feel anything in the face of their child's illness, like Katie:

"How are you feeling?"

"I'm okay. Rachael's had another transfusion which seems to have given her a little more energy and her sickness following chemo was manageable this time. The skin around her stoma's sore and she's had to have three new NG tubes passed..."

"Okay. So that's Rachael. But I asked how you are doing?"

"Oh. Well, in that case, I'm feeling guilty because I have been away from Henry – he's only just three, he doesn't understand what's happening. I'm feeling guilty that I have no energy left to support my husband. I feel isolated because I've built up barriers. I don't want help. I want all the help to be directed towards Rachael – whose medical need is overwhelming – and towards my family, who need more help and support than I can provide."

I wouldn't even have engaged with the counselling offered on the paediatric oncology ward if I hadn't been told it would support my daughter's treatment. When you have a child who is seriously ill you don't want to think about how you're doing. How you're doing is not a priority.

So how does childhood illness make parents feel? Empty. Numb. Too guilty to feel. Childhood illness has the freezing effect of trauma. Childhood illness makes parents stop feeling.

That is what happened to me when my daughter was born. I stopped feeling. I froze in the face of flashing lights, screeching alarms, masked doctors and nurses surrounding her tiny body, wires, tubes, monitors. An ambulance sent to rush her away – unaccompanied, because of Covid restrictions. A Neonatal Intensive Care cot. A cot to protect her... but from what? From me. From my instinct to grab her and run. It was devastating heartbreak for what she had to go through. Devastation at the discovery of so many tumours and diagnosis of a rare condition that could only be treated with chemotherapy. Devastating survival rates, heartbreakingly low. But as well as the heart-stopping trauma there was a miraculous flicker, a ground-breaking and life-saving path back to feeling. Desperate hope.

That desperate hope gave me a tether back to my feelings. And, at first, I had to physically cling on to those feelings: as much skin-to-skin with my daughter as I could get, holding her at my breast even when she was too poorly to latch; hugging my son so tightly I could breathe him in; clasping at my husband's hand as we sat through consultations.

Slowly, I began to see the path back, navigating the practicalities of treatments, feeding, sleep, side-effects, surgeries, scans, frequent and lengthy hospital stays. Frozen with trauma, I just had to live through it.

But living through it wasn't enough. Increasingly, I came to realise that I needed to love through it. I needed to be able to feel love. Feeling is what makes us human. Feeling love for our children is what makes us parents. And, whatever the future holds, love is the answer. For our blessings – love is joy and gratitude. For our grief – love lasts – beyond pain, beyond loss, beyond everything.'

<u>Catherine Young</u>

Why Childhood Illness Matters

While it is inappropriate to equate the suffering of sick children with that of parents, it is understandable that loving parents would be hurt by the experience of caring for their sick child. In the essential work of supporting sick children, we must never forget that parents need care and attention too.

Not what they planned

When a parent first sees that blue line on a pregnancy test, they imagine a life for their child that is largely free of illness. Nobody ever chooses to parent in the hospital setting. It is different, frightening and exposed. There is very little privacy in what would otherwise be a personal experience of parenting. Everyone expects to give birth, hold their baby, take their baby home, and raise their child, with the usual ups and downs, but no major catastrophe.

Parents all around the world today will be having prenatal scans – of course, it's normal to worry that the scan will reveal something unusual or worrying, but most people are mainly looking forward to seeing their wriggly unborn baby, and the biggest drama is usually deciding whether to find out the baby's sex or not. For a small number of parents, this is where their visions of a perfect childhood become altered beyond recognition. The talk turns to neonatal intensive care units, surgery or intense medical treatments.

Some parents are blindsided by a sudden onset of illness, and other children go back and forth to various medical professionals in a parent's fiercely determined search for the root cause of a problem that has slowly revealed itself.

> *'Hirschprung's, as with so many complex diagnoses, has so much more to it than meets the eye. When expecting your first child, you never imagine signing consent forms for surgery from a few days old or holding them as they*

are put under anaesthetic for nine hours, scalp cannulas or Hickman lines, being faced with getting air-lifted from your holiday, with only a Facebook group of families all experiencing their own crises as any sort of peer support.

Going through something like this changes you and sets you apart – it can be hard to connect to some other parents as they navigate their own challenges, which feel so trivial in comparison. Approaching another pregnancy with the awareness that you have an increased risk, even if relatively low, of going through all the trauma again is emotionally wearing.' Hannah Maillardet

Whatever a child's condition, whether it was diagnosed before birth, in the first few days, or several months or years later – this is not an easy path to walk. Parents have to develop a 'new normal'. Redefine their expectations. Change their plans. Indeed, an early lesson in childhood illness is to hold on to plans lightly, being prepared to drop them, or change them. Over time, this can build resilience, humour, flexibility and spontaneity, but this shift towards making the best of it takes time.

Another obvious point perhaps, but it's okay for parents to acknowledge that their child's hospitalisation is a major disappointment, inconvenience and frustration to them on a personal level, even though their primary concern is for their child on a more altruistic level. They don't have to be happy about the situation. A parent may spend their *own* birthday, anniversary or special holiday in hospital. They may miss events, occasions and holidays due to childhood illness. Their career may take a hit. It's normal to feel disappointed and angry about these realities.

A balance between redefining the new normal and maintaining life as parents knew it may be important for their emotional wellbeing. Many parents experience a blinding panic that they suddenly need to change everything. They may find themselves at 2am scouring property websites, convinced that they will need to move house to a single-level building. Their mind may leap ahead to researching schools with excellent special educational needs provision. They might draft their resignation letter for their employer at work. But before they do any or all these things, it's usually a good idea to just *pause*. Some situations will of course require adaptations, but this does not mean their whole life has to be immediately turned upside-down.

The disruption to normality

The impacts on childhood and family life of frequent or long-term hospitalisation are far reaching. It helps to be aware of the possible disruptions parents and families may face along the way. You might not be able to prevent all frustrations or disappointments, but preparation means less drama and anxiety. In fact, some research has found that it is the disruption to normal activities of daily living that causes the most distress, rather than the uncertainty of diagnosis. One study exploring the stressors experienced by children with a cancer diagnosis and their parents found that both children and parents found the disruption to normal life more stressful than the diagnosis itself (Rodriguez et al, 2012). This study also found that parental stress was significantly higher with younger children (aged five and younger) than with children aged 5–10 years. This was mainly due to the uncontrollability of some of the aspects of caregiving. Obviously, as children get older, they become more independent and begin to take more responsibility for their health. Younger children are much more likely to need more physical care, as well as having reduced capacity to understand the disruption to normal life

– such as hospitalisation, isolation, treatments, medication, investigations and so on.

There is also some evidence that parenting behaviours may be affected by childhood illness. One of the most obvious ways that this can happen is that during certain periods of illness, it is absolutely appropriate that a sick child may need their parents' emotional support more, require greater parental input (especially for very young children) or more physical help. However, this can subtly spill over into other areas where they do not need as much help (Pinquart, 2013). It can require a conscious effort not to over-protect children and get the balance right.

Trauma

There is plentiful literature relating to the impact of childhood illness and hospitalisation on families. One qualitative study found that both children and parents reported shock, sadness, confusion, frustration, and anger. Parents additionally experience feelings of numbness and worry (Gannoni and Shute, 2010). Stress, trauma and anxiety are also frequently described by parents (Mortensen et al., 2015; Muscara et al., 2015; Foster et al., 2017) and other research recommends that parents are provided with adequate psychological support during hospitalisation of their child for a life-threatening condition (Smith et al., 2015; Pelentsov et al., 2015). Some parents develop post-traumatic stress disorder after watching their child becoming profoundly unwell, witnessing their child's resuscitation, or receiving a diagnosis of a life-threatening disease or condition (Woolf et al., 2016).

'For families who spend long periods of time in hospital or who like us are "frequent flyers", psychological support is key. It took much longer than it really should

have for me to realise that I had post-traumatic stress disorder because of the many medical interventions and hospital admissions Reuben has had. It didn't come as a surprise to the specialists I eventually spoke to and I feel strongly that even if it is not possible to pre-emptively offer psychological support to everyone, certainly at least speaking to families to give them an awareness that they are more at risk of developing mental health problems and an awareness of the symptoms to look out for, might mean that they are able to recognise it and seek help at an earlier stage.' Gemma Nixon

No one form of therapy will work equally for all parents in all situations. Cognitive behavioural therapy has been shown to work well for some parents of children with medical complexity (Law et al., 2019), but for other families, diaries (McIlroy et al., 2019), or eye movement desensitisation and reprocessing (EMDR) work better (Dominguez et al., 2021).

The psychological journey of diagnosis

'It was 5am on an August bank holiday weekend when my firstborn baby boy had his first seizure at just eight weeks old. After days in intensive care, the doctors sat me and my husband down on a sofa in a private room with a box of tissues on the table. They looked at us with sombre expressions and tilted heads. We both knew something was deeply wrong.

After what felt like endless small talk, they broke the news to us that an MRI scan had found that our son had bilateral perisylvian polymicrogyria. They told us it was a neurological condition that meant his brain structure was different. They told us that some people with this

condition couldn't swallow, some didn't have any mobility, the chance of intellectual disability was very high, many had epilepsy (which our son now has), and a host of other medical conditions. The symptoms and limitations they described were specific, and the reassurances they offered were vague and faded into the background.

Through therapy, I now know that I experienced "dissociation": one part of me went into autopilot, asking thoughtful questions and making detailed notes. Simultaneously, another part of me (that no one could see) fell to her knees and screamed into a vast darkness. I saw my world shatter into a billion tiny fragments. My dreams were devastated. My hopes were crushed. Every door of opportunity slammed shut. Fear clouded everything. It has taken therapy and years of healing to repair the wound that the moment of our son's diagnosis created within me.' Shurron Rosales

Ways of coping

I've seen people deploy different types of coping strategy during the stress and upheaval of diagnosis and serious illness. We all have an automatic stress response, over which we have little control. This includes our physical reaction to stress – such as sweaty palms, racing heart, nausea, loss of appetite and so on. It also encompasses some of the automatic emotional processes, such as panic, irrational thoughts and behaving as if on 'auto-pilot'. In this state, people may find that they do procedural tasks without even realising what they have done. Others may pace the floor or tap their foot. We can't always control these types of behaviour.

Stress and anxiety feel exhausting from a physiological point of view. A stressed body and mind are working hard, and many parents feel that their usual stress coping strategies simply do not work. They may attempt to read a book to distract themselves, only to find that they read the same sentence 17 times because they cannot focus. They may eat more, feel nauseous, or find it impossible to sleep.

But we also develop intentional coping mechanisms. Parents may need to pull out different strategies at different times, or they may have a go-to strategy that they default to. Coping mechanisms may be problem-focused or emotion-focused; proactive or avoidant; passive or active. For example, some parents may go on an internet-fuelled mission to find out everything they can about their child's condition (problem-focused). Or they might throw themselves into journaling (emotion focused). They could take up knitting, crochet or colouring (distraction), or utilise the power of positive thinking (Compas et al., 2012). Other parents call a friend or family member, pray, focus on their breath, or meditate. While reading may feel impossible, listening to music, an audiobook or podcast might be worth trying.

For some parents, bustling around making plans is a coping mechanism. Others throw themselves into a project. I wrote my first book largely at my daughter's bedside, whiling away those long evenings in hospital isolation rooms – it was both a focus and a distraction. There are many adaptations to a stressful situation. Parents need to find the one that's right for them, their situation and their stress response. While nothing works for absolutely everyone, many parents may appreciate some suggestions.

2
Types of illness

Clearly it would be impractical to list every single childhood illness. We'd be here all day and I still might miss out the one condition that the child you are supporting happens to have. What I've done instead is split illnesses into acute, chronic and lifelong categories as they all present unique challenges.

Acute illnesses include coughs and colds, and you might quite reasonably wonder at first glance why I've included these at all. The main reason is that children with chronic and lifelong illnesses *also* suffer from acute and self-limiting illnesses and infections. The second is that I never want to trivialise anyone's experience of ill-health. Children being ill is never fabulous, let's face it. Whatever parents are facing with their child is significant, and it is likely that many children will inevitably segue between acute and chronic illness.

Acute illness

If a child has an acute illness or infection, this means that they become unwell suddenly, and it is usually something that is short in duration. Occasionally the word gets confusing, as it can be erroneously thought of as 'minor'. But anyone who has known someone with an acute myocardial infarction, or acute trauma, or acute lymphoblastic leukaemia knows that this is not necessarily the case at all. The word 'acute' is simply used to differentiate it from a more chronic form of a similar illness.

Acute conditions can come on out of seemingly nowhere. You'll know this yourself. Hands up who's had an acute gastrointestinal upset? In the morning you're fine, by lunchtime… uh-oh! They're rapid in their onset, but they are not necessarily minor, as I will explain. It may be that you are supporting a family at home when you become concerned about the health of a child and need to recommend that they seek urgent medical care. Unless the child also has an arrangement with the local ward for rapid access, acute infections that require medical attention will usually pass through the accident and emergency department.

Accident & Emergency (A&E)

If a child has a condition that can't be managed at home, or if they have an underlying condition which necessitates more caution with illnesses, they will experience A&E. Not all hospitals have an A&E department. Some just have a minor injury unit or have restrictions and limits on their capacity to see younger children, so if in doubt, call first, or ring 111 to ask for advice. Almost all hospitals that *do* have an A&E will have a paediatric section, though the size and whether this is staffed 24/7 may vary. In most cases, there will be a separate paediatric waiting area, with paediatric-trained staff, more child-friendly décor, children's toys and furniture, and so on. Paediatric A&E still has all the emergency equipment you would expect from an emergency facility, including resus

Types of illness

bays and isolation areas for infectious conditions.

First, a nurse will triage a child. They will take a brief history and do a set of clinical observations – temperature, pulse, oxygen saturations, respiratory rate, blood pressure, and sometimes a capillary refill, blood sugar, Glasgow coma scale if there is a head injury, and pain score to assess their condition and the seriousness of the situation. After this, depending on their initial assessment, just like in any other A&E department, the parents and their child will either be immediately treated if their condition warrants, or wait in turn to be seen and further assessed and treated by a nurse practitioner, GP or paediatrician as appropriate. How long they will wait is dependent on how many other children there are, how seriously ill the child is, and how seriously unwell *other* children are.

When the child is seen, the assessing clinician will make a judgement call about whether they need:

- urgent stablisation or resuscitation
- immediate tests – such as an X-ray, scans or a blood test
- assessment by another member of staff – such as a senior colleague, or a colleague with a specific specialism, like ENT, plastics or the surgical team
- immediate treatment – such as antibiotics, a plaster cast or stitches
- escalation to more intensive treatment – such as a transfer to a hospital that can provide high-dependency or intensive paediatric care.

There is also a decision to be made about whether the child can be given treatment in the A&E department and then sent home, or whether they need to be admitted to this hospital (or transferred to another one). Whatever the outcome, parents should ensure they understand what is going on, and if they have questions about how the clinicians are making their decisions, they can always ask. For example, if they make the decision *not* to admit a child, but a parent remains worried, it's okay for them to explain their concerns and ensure that they are clear about why the doctors have made that decision.

Self-limiting illness

This is a bizarre phrase (in my humble opinion!). Not many people outside the clinical world understand what it means, despite the regularity with which it is used. This term basically means that whatever the child has will go away on its own, without any special treatment. This applies to many minor viral illnesses including coughs and colds, tummy bugs, ear infections and all manner of nastiness that children are prone to contracting in their first few years. It means that medicines such as antibiotics, or any other interventions, are not required for the illness to get better. This does not mean that the illness isn't horrible, inconvenient or upsetting – it just means that apart from basic pain relief (if appropriate and safe to give), and TLC (tender loving care), there isn't anything anyone can do. Obviously, while it is still frustrating to have to deal with illness, this is reassuring. However, it certainly does not mean that you were wrong to access a medical opinion. It is *always* appropriate to refer to a clinician if you are unsure about the severity of an illness. It is not a parent or a non-clinician's job to diagnose or clinically assess a child – it is only their responsibility to refer to the person who *can*.

Paediatric clinicians would always rather see a child too early than too late. Never, ever worry that you're wasting anyone's time.

Occasionally, if a child has an underlying condition, an illness that would be self-limiting for most children can be more serious. For example, for most children chicken pox is an annoying inconvenience. But for an immunocompromised child it can be serious, and this means that they will require more treatment than other children. At other times children with an underlying condition will be treated very cautiously because there isn't time to figure out exactly what illness they have. For example, children being treated for cancer will be overtreated for many self-limiting conditions. It isn't sensible to pontificate about whether the illness is a serious central line infection or just a cough and cold, so they are likely to be treated as intensively as a child with sepsis would be. The bottom line is that how the child is treated for a self-limiting condition will depend on the context of their health history.

Brief but serious acute illness

Acute illnesses can be very serious. One child can have tonsillitis that is self-limiting, while another will become overwhelmingly unwell and require more intensive treatment. One tummy bug will be a minor inconvenience, while another may require fluid resuscitation. Some meningitis infections require only observation and supportive treatment, while others require intensive care. Many illnesses have a spectrum of severity of presentation. Again, acute does not mean 'minor'!

If a child suddenly becomes very unwell, it can be very shocking for those caring for them. It's not unusual to hear that a child was 'fine' in the morning and by bedtime was having emergency surgery for appendicitis. Or what was thought to be a cough and cold that seemed minor can take a rapid turn for the worse and lead to hospital admission.

The bottom line with these 'zero to 60' illnesses is to trust your gut instinct and get help as soon as possible. I've never met a paediatric clinician who would rather parents did not bring in a child they were worried about. It's always better to get them checked and be sent home than to worry. Yes, hospitals are busy places and staff are overstretched, but this is literally what they're there for.

We will come back to how these very serious and rapid illnesses can affect families later in Chapter 6, but for now, suffice it to say that these experiences can be very traumatic. There's something about the rapid deterioration of usually vibrant children that feels a bit like psychological whiplash. As well as ensuring the parent has support, these experiences can be distressing for anyone else caring for young children, so try to debrief with a friend or colleague if you can. Supervision relevant to the role you are working in is incredibly important to maintain professionalism, as well as maintain safety and appropriate boundaries. If you are on the ward with your child or the child you care for, please make sure you take care of yourself – remember to eat, even if you just nibble on small snacks. My wise Dad always says 'If you can't eat calories, drink calories' – and I can't tell you how often I have had to resort to smoothies and juices because I can't force food down! Leaving the ward for short breaks also helps – so try to swap with someone to get a rest if you can.

Acute on chronic

Some more jargon for you! This means an acute exacerbation of a known chronic condition. For example, some children have asthma which is normally managed with regular inhalers, but have asthma attacks requiring more frequent or continuous treatment. Many chronic conditions can flare up from time to time. A child may need admission to the ward during one of these acute flare-ups, which can feel worrying and frustrating if their condition is normally managed at home. It's also hard not to worry about whether this was something that could have been prevented, or something that could happen again.

Types of illness

All of these are rational fears. While it's easy to say, 'try not to worry about what's not under your control', the reality is that it's hard to do.

If a child is getting more frequent acute on chronic illnesses or flare-ups of their condition it may be that their treatment and management plan needs reviewing, which the doctors in charge of the child's condition will arrange. Perhaps their medication needs adjusting or increasing, or maybe there is a new problem. It may help if you keep a symptom diary to track whether there is an obvious trigger or environmental cause for the flare-ups.

Chronic illness

Chronic illnesses are generally defined as those that last more than three months. Of these, some may be lifelong conditions, such as diabetes, cystic fibrosis, sickle cell anaemia, and coeliac disease, while others may cause health problems for some time until the treatment has been completed – such as cancer, and some congenital conditions that can be managed with surgery. Chronic illness is sometimes diagnosed before or soon after birth. Sometimes a chronic illness sneaks up on your child. Other times it occurs because of an acute infection. For some children, the diagnosis is uncertain. Many chronic illnesses have periods of relapse and remission – when their condition flares up requiring more intense treatment, followed by a period when the condition is stable. While I almost certainly cannot do justice to every permutation of chronic childhood illness, I'll group experiences to help you find the support you need.

Prematurity

Chronologically, the first time point to consider is prematurity.

Infants who are born before 37 weeks of pregnancy are defined as preterm:

- *Extremely preterm*   less than 28 weeks
- *Very preterm*   28–32 weeks
- *Moderately preterm*   32–37 weeks

Preterm babies are not a homogenous group, and their prematurity is not necessarily correlated with how unwell they are or how much support they will need. A baby born at 36 weeks may need more intensive treatment than a baby born at 34 weeks, depending on multiple factors, including underlying conditions. However, in general, the more preterm a baby, the more likely they are to need intensive care.

Premature babies may need weeks or months of treatment and support to be well enough to go home, but this does not necessarily mean that they will have additional chronic conditions because of their prematurity. Every child and family's experience is unique.

If you are supporting the family of a premature infant, all their clinical care will be delivered by a specialist neonatal team and it's important to remember scope of practice here. What works for healthy term infants does not necessarily work for preterm infants, and these families are often also dealing with complex clinical needs and trauma as well. Make sure you check what a family has been told by the neonatal team to avoid contradictory or confusing messages. Once they are discharged, all queries about ongoing health, oxygen or feeding needs can be directed to the neonatal outreach teams.

Types of illness

The perspective of a specialist neonatal nurse

Having worked across the spectrum of neonatal care, i.e., NICU, high dependency, special care, transitional care, and community care (neonatal outreach), I have seen how valuable the wider support team can be for families whose babies require the support of an admission into neonatal care. In my experience as a neonatal outreach nurse and infant feeding lead, I have found it so rewarding to lead on managing faltering growth in the community, which includes:

- Having an understanding of monitoring trends
- How to take measurements accurately
- The best way to plot these measurements (hint: it is probably worth using a close monitoring growth chart to see trends more easily without the 'actual age' and 'correcting' charting taking up space)
- Understanding the treatment and monitoring aims
- Knowing when to update and ask for guidance from allied healthcare professionals.

And obviously all this is alongside aiming to meet feeding goals. Despite learning acquired from courses, study days, and my own review of material, it is essential that I work closely with a specialist dietitian to ensure that care is up to date, accurate, and relevant. I have had the privilege of seeing families and their babies thrive when messages and communication are consistent, with those in support roles liaising appropriately with those with specialist training and the remit to create and deliver care. A neonatal service without an infant feeding lead nurse may liaise with the parent's independent IBCLC or the infant feeding team in maternity, for example, putting their specialist knowledge together to create an individualised package of care that is appropriate for that baby and family.

It is important to remember that, wherever a family may be within neonatal care, e.g. whether a mother is getting to know her newborn 24-weeker, starting to introduce breastfeeding on the neonatal unit for a baby that is now 34 weeks corrected gestational age, weaning from oxygen at home for their ex-30-weeker, weaning from tube feeds and continuing to establish oral feeds at home for their 35-weeker that was born to a mother with gestational diabetes, and so on, they continue to require neonatal input from professionals that have extensive underpinning knowledge and experience of *this* baby's journey and those similar because of their needs at that time. Inappropriately making decisions or recommendations outside professional remit, introducing conflict in care plans, and a multidisciplinary team that works against one another leaves families confused and frustrated at best and babies receiving delayed input and treatment with increased morbidity and mortality at worst. Instead, if there is disagreement, try to work together to build understanding and enhance bespoke care.

Amanda Smith, *paediatric nurse, qualified neonatal nurse and IBCLC*

Antenatal diagnosis

If a child is diagnosed with a condition antenatally the family may have some time to prepare for any additional health needs that they may have. The child may be admitted straight to the

Types of illness

neonatal unit if their condition means they require immediate support – such as certain cardiac defects, airway problems or major gastrointestinal anomalies. Other children may be observed on the postnatal ward to ensure that they are feeding and growing well – for instance if they have a condition that does not require immediate treatment.

Antenatal diagnosis can be a huge shock, and many parents may find themselves feeling angry, upset or confused. They may find that a visit to the neonatal unit – if their child is likely to be cared for there – will alleviate some of the anxiety of the unknown. Many parents also throw themselves into learning about their child's condition so they can be prepared. Joining support groups for parents with children who have the same condition can be a great way of getting some much-needed peer support from people who have walked a similar path. If you are involved with families of children with complex needs from the start you may also find it helpful to find out as much as possible beforehand.

Perinatal and later diagnosis

For many families, a diagnosis of chronic illness is made following obvious problems that arise after birth, often with the way a child feeds or behaves, their muscle tone or bodily function. For some families, chronic illnesses arise after an apparently healthy few months or years, such as diabetes and epilepsy. It can be devastating to see a normally bouncy child flattened by ill-health. Some of these illnesses and conditions require long or multiple periods of hospitalisation, surgery and outpatient appointments.

Roisin's daughter was diagnosed with acute myeloid leukaemia (AML) at four months:

'My daughter Aila was born healthy with no complications at birth. At about four weeks old, like all of us, she caught a cold, and I started to notice that while everyone else recovered, she wasn't getting better. We started to visit the GP and our local hospital multiple times, each one giving us no answers. She was tiny, unable to gain any weight, struggling to breathe, had bruised lumps on her head, her eyes were protruding, she could sleep 20 hours a day and she was incredibly upset and hard to settle. I was told how lucky I was to have a baby that slept so much, but I knew that it was something else.

Several months later, after persistently asking to be seen, we saw an amazing consultant who really took the time to listen to me and sent us for bloods. Three hours after the bloods were taken, I got a call asking us to bring Aila back to hospital with an overnight bag. Immediately I knew it was cancer, and we rushed in. As soon as we got there two consultants were waiting for us; this was a bad sign. I don't remember much from that conversation, but they told us "to take a seat together, we were about to have a conversation we would never forget". "Aila has leukaemia, and we need to urgently transfer her to a specialist hospital". That night I felt like grief had hit me, I had lost this beautiful healthy baby and our life as we knew it was shattered.

We stayed in our local hospital that night as we waited for an intensive care bed at a specialist oncology hospital. Aila rapidly declined overnight as they started to give her medication in a desperate attempt to protect her organs. The night was never-ending, and I remember vomiting outside the hospital as my body was in shock.

A specialist intensive care children's ambulance collected us and placed Aila into a portable intensive

Types of illness

care pod. We were told Aila was so unwell they didn't know if she would survive the 40-minute drive to the next hospital, and that at any point we might need to pull over for her to be resuscitated. Once we arrived, they stabilised her in intensive care and sedated her. We were told to bring our families up to say goodbye, because things were not looking great.

We spent five days in intensive care, with countless tests, and they kept her intubated the whole time. Her organs were starting to fail, and she was at risk of life-threatening seizures. The bad news kept coming, they told us she had tumours all across her skull and that she was too unwell to start chemotherapy yet. But Aila is a fighter, and finally she was diagnosed with acute myeloid leukaemia a day before she turned five months. A rare leukaemia in such a young baby, and one that came with very intense chemotherapy.

We were transferred to the oncology ward where she immediately began chemotherapy. We signed consent forms for chemotherapy that listed all the horrible side-effects that our daughter had no choice but to go through. Our treatment plan was four courses of chemo, each 10 days of chemo followed by six weeks of rest, all as an inpatient. She would become too immune-compromised to be able to even leave her room.

Her strength was incredible, she battled many infections including sepsis which she required emergency surgery for. Aila had her last chemotherapy on Christmas morning and has reached remission. She rang her end of treatment bell and is now thriving at home. Finally, we can walk in the fresh air, our families and friends can get to know her, she can play and enjoy life.' Roisin Butler

Supporting families of children with chronic illness

Some chronic illnesses can be treated, while other children have conditions that they must learn to live with – such as asthma, diabetes, sickle cell disease and cystic fibrosis. It is impossible to do justice to the huge variety of conditions with which a child may be diagnosed, so I will focus instead on some of the reported challenges in general of this group of families and how you can support them. The needs of children with profound medical complexity are covered in Chapter 6.

While many chronic illnesses and conditions may be manageable, they are worrying, disruptive and require vigilance to monitor a child's condition. Some children can be managed with medication, while others need no regular medication until they experience a flare-up of their condition. The long-term nature of chronic illness can be difficult for parents and children alike – it is common for them to experience anger, frustration and anxiety. Therefore, one of the areas of support that a family may need to access is psychological and talking therapies. Addressing the 'why me/my child' type of questions is arguably part of the process of accepting a childhood or lifelong condition. There is often a psychologist based in the paediatric department to whom families can be referred, but it is worth checking what services are available. Some families may opt to access private support, which may offer them more flexibility and timely access to care. Above all, allowing families the time to talk in the way that is helpful for them is very cathartic. Sometimes just having someone listen is the best type of therapy.

One of the challenges of parenting children with long-term health conditions is the balance of maintaining boundaries and limits, while also making appropriate allowances at times because of the nature of their illness or condition. For example, it is entirely understandable that a child might scream and shout about having to have another blood test, but it is not appropriate to ignore that child hitting their sibling in their frustration. Many parents have a conversation about what their boundaries are irrespective of the child's condition, and decide whether there are any sensible exceptions or adaptations that need to be made, either due to cognitive understanding, pain or hospitalisation. Essentially – boundaries are still required, but are there ever circumstances in which the boundaries need to flex?

Finally, children with chronic illness are often tough, and become experts on their own health needs and their condition. But they still need to be allowed to be children, build their self-esteem, socialise with other children, and not become defined by their condition. There may be a balance to find where the child is empowered with the information they need about their condition and treatment, but does not take on too much age-inappropriate responsibility for it. This is hard to get right, but the specialist nurses the child is likely to have access to are usually really good at providing information in a child-centred way and involving other professionals when necessary. It's also important to allow children to have normal experiences and opportunities if it is safe and appropriate to do so. It can be tempting to wrap them in cotton wool, but this may not be in their best interests.

> *'My son has Von Willebrand disease, which is a clotting disorder. When we first found out we were terrified he would fall over in the playground and have a catastrophic bleed. Every instinct was to keep him off school to protect him. But I slowly realised that he couldn't effectively be "off sick" for most of his childhood. I was scared, but we had a helpful talk with the haematologist and then the school nurse about what we could do to keep him safe but*

still let him be a little boy. We decided that contact sports were off the table, but there was no reason for him to avoid most other lessons. The school nurse knows about his condition, and he has an alert in the office.' <u>Michelle Taylor</u>

Supporting children with chronic illness requires more planning, creativity and an understanding that plans will need to evolve with age and changes in condition. But with the right expertise and carefully curated care plans many children can be helped to access some or all of the usual activities of childhood.

3
On the ward

For most parents of children with illness or medical complexity, hospital will be a part of life to a greater or lesser extent. While no book can change the fact that being in hospital even once, never mind several times, is hugely disruptive and distressing, hopefully knowing who everyone is and what their role is will enable families to feel more confident in this very strange environment. It's also important to know about the variety of professional roles so that families know who to speak to for further advice and support.

People families might meet

Perhaps you have experienced hospital hierarchies, or maybe you've been cared for in a hospital that is more egalitarian. But either way, to avoid this looking like any one member of the team is more or less 'important', these are the people you're likely to meet, and what their role is, in alphabetical order:

Administrative staff

Families will meet a variety of admin staff – including the

ward clerk, receptionists, medical records staff, secretaries and appointment clerks. They put up with a massive amount of nonsense and often have the patience of saints. They're there to make sure everything runs smoothly from an administrative point of view, and you may also communicate with them to make and rearrange appointments or chase up test results.

Catering team

It's not easy managing the food for thousands of patients with multiple different cultural, dietary and religious food preferences. Catering often comes under fire when people criticise the health service, but I have huge sympathy for the gargantuan task that it must be. Heck – it's hard enough to create a nutritious meal for a small family! All that said, I know that sometimes food can be a real bone of contention if there aren't good options. For instance, if the only dinner option for a vegan who is also a coeliac and needs a gluten-free option is a salad, someone's going to go hungry, so please do provide feedback if the options don't meet the needs of families. But don't give the serving staff a hard time – it's definitely not their fault.

Chaplaincy team

There is often a multi-faith chaplaincy team, or there may be a representative from a particular faith group based in the hospital. There may also be a multi-faith prayer room that anyone can use for quiet contemplation or to speak to a member of the chaplaincy staff. The chaplains will make time to talk to parents and may call into the wards from time to time, but do not usually do a standard 'ward round', so ask the nurse caring for the child to bleep them if you, or your child, would like to talk to them.

On the ward

Healthcare assistants and nursery nurses

HCAs are important non-clinical members of staff who work alongside the clinical team, often closely with a nurse. They support the nursing staff by taking on tasks such as clinical observations (checking a child's temperature, pulse, respiratory rate and so on). They may also weigh and measure children in outpatients, and support children with eating, drinking and moving around. Some HCAs have a dual role as a phlebotomist as well. Nursery nurses are also not clinically trained, but have a valuable role supporting children, encouraging their normal development, maintaining a child-friendly environment and providing hands-on care of children. They may undertake some more clinical roles, such as giving feeds or doing clinical observations under the supervision of a registered nurse.

Housekeeping staff

You'll often find that the people you see most regularly are the housekeeping staff. While nursing shifts are all over the place, families will often see the same housekeeper most days, and they can frequently be a cheery and kind face as well as helping to keep the ward tidy, fresh and clean.

Infant feeding lead and team

There is usually no designated paediatric infant feeding lead or team. However, as Baby Friendly Standards begin to be embedded in paediatric wards and children's hospitals, my hope is that increasingly, infant feeding teams with paediatric training will be trained in the specific nuanced feeding needs of older infants and children, as well as the feeding challenges of children with a diverse range of conditions. In the meantime, if a child requires feeding support, the staff may be able to ask the maternity or neonatal infant feeding team to come to see a family. These professionals may also be able to source breastpumps and other equipment.

Nurses

Every child will be allocated a paediatric nurse who will oversee all their care, including supervising any care provided by an HCA. The nurse will provide a child's medication, IV fluids, do certain procedures, check clinical observations, liaise between the doctors and families, accompany children on transfers to other hospitals, and supervise and arrange any tests and transport needed. They will also be the ones checking on a child's condition and alerting the right members of staff if there is a change. Nurses usually work on just one ward, so it's likely that families will get to know many familiar faces, though shift patterns may mean they see one nurse for three days straight, and then don't see them again for a week. There are also specialist nurses who have clinical condition-specific expertise, who may be involved with a child's care, and may see them in clinic, or provide additional advice to general paediatric nurses. Parents may also have contact with the nurse in charge – usually a more experienced nurse who will have their own patients to look after but will also supervise the shift. Finally, there is a ward manager, charge nurse or matron who usually does not have a clinical caseload and has more of a managerial role, though they will be very clinically experienced.

Paediatricians

A paediatrician is the doctor in charge of the child's overall care and management plan. They assess, diagnose and treat children in all paediatric areas, so unlike nurses, they do not only care for a small number of patients on one ward, but have responsibility for many children, including those who are seen in the emergency department. They divide their time between the wards, operating theatres, outpatient clinics and the emergency department. There is likely to be a named paediatrician looking after a child's care, but this does not mean the family will see only them. They work in teams and have on-call patterns so families might not necessarily see them every day. Paediatricians will establish a diagnosis, and then work up a management plan with any tests or procedures based on that diagnosis. They then delegate some of those tests or procedures to nursing staff, therapists or other doctors. Families will usually see a doctor every day while in hospital when they do their 'ward round' (more on this later).

Pharmacists

Pharmacists are there to oversee the prescribing, usage, dispensing and administration of drugs in the hospital. They work on the ward, and in the hospital dispensary and the hospital outpatient pharmacy. They may offer advice to clinicians about drug interactions and allergies, or make suggestions for the correct treatment depending on blood or specimen culture results. They also work with dietitians to support the prescription of total parenteral nutrition (TPN). They're also involved in audit, risk and safety management of drugs, and oversee drug and clinical trials requiring specific medications.

Phlebotomists

Phlebotomists are specially trained members of staff who are experts in taking blood and may also site cannulas – though in some hospitals, cannulation is the exclusive realm of those who are medically trained. Many of the clinicians families will meet can do these roles, including nurses and doctors, but phlebotomists are usually fantastic as they do this all day long and have lots of experience with even the trickiest veins! They may surprise you by not choosing the most obvious, bouncy vein, but going for a more obscure spot. Trust them – they not only know which veins are likely to be more successful to cannulate, but also which ones are more precarious and likely to fall out. Of course, some people are just harder to cannulate and take blood from than others, and I have enormous respect for these professionals who are magicians at this job.

Play specialists

Play is a fundamental right of childhood and is important for social and emotional development as well as learning. Hospitals are scary places for children and play specialists are experts in child development and communication (Perasso et al., 2021). They use a combination of normal play, distraction, and medical play. Normal play is obviously provided to support a child's social and emotional development, so they do not miss out on these opportunities. Distraction is a key technique during certain procedures and can be as effective as pharmacological pain relief. And medical play is the deliberate use of toys, puppets, or objects to prepare children for a specific procedure. Play *specialists* are different from play *therapists*, who use counselling techniques as part of psychotherapy. A child or their sibling may be separately referred to a play therapist for specific purposes, such as to work through some of their feelings about childhood illness.

Porters

Porters are crucial within hospitals. These under-appreciated wonderful people move patients first and foremost, but also equipment, linen, samples and furniture around the hospital as needed. If a child needs an X-ray, scan, or has to go to the operating theatre, you'll meet a porter. If a little one gets transferred to another ward – you need a porter. If a baby requires an urgent blood transfusion, a porter may run the bloods to the lab for cross-matching. I've met porters who are speedy sprinters, porters who dress up to cheer the kids up, and porters who make patients (old and young) laugh. I have no idea what we'd do without them.

Psychotherapists

Some units, especially specialist units, have a counsellor or psychologist attached to the ward. Parents or children (and sometimes both) may be able to access them to talk through how they are feeling and coping. In many cases, this can be a lot faster than waiting for a referral via a GP, plus these staff are very experienced at supporting parents through the complex emotional and psychological issues surrounding childhood illness. It is not any kind of weakness or evidence that you are 'not coping' to talk to someone. If you feel it would be helpful, please access this service.

Radiologists and radiographers

If a child needs an imaging scan, this will be performed by a radiographer. Radiographers are allied health professionals who position children for their scans, undertake the scan and are skilled in getting the right images. Radiologists are doctors who have additional training and specialism in performing interventions under guided imaging, as well as interpreting images to make a diagnosis or assessment. If you have ever seen an ultrasound, CT, MRI or X-ray image you may have marvelled at the skill of those who can diagnose conditions or pathology by looking at the image, which may look like a grey, black and white blob to the untrained eye!

Social workers

There will be a social worker attached to the ward to whom

the staff can refer families. Social workers do a variety of jobs – please do not think that if a family has been referred to one that the hospital staff are concerned about the child's welfare from a safeguarding point of view. Social workers often become involved when children have complex needs, to ensure that families have access to all the support they need. They may assist with helping them apply for benefits, or disability living allowance, or organise the delivery of home-based support. They will often liaise with different professionals and generally be there as the parents' (and the child's) advocate.

Students

All clinicians have to learn, and families are almost guaranteed to meet nursing, allied health and medical students on the ward at some point. Student nurses will usually shadow a nursing 'mentor', but depending on what stage they are at in their training, families may see more or less of the student. They will usually be differentiated by uniform, and their name badge will also clearly state that they are a student. If you're ever unsure, you can always ask the child's nurse. You may also see medical and allied health professional students – they will usually be under the direct supervision of a clinician.

Teachers

If a child is under the age of five years, they won't have a lot to do with the hospital teaching staff. But for those children over five, who would usually be in school during the week, the teachers provide an invaluable link to normality, as well as providing a distraction and preventing a child's learning journey from being derailed by illness. Of course, children do not *have* to participate in school while they are in hospital – this is an offer, not a requirement. If they're too unwell, tired,

On the ward

or do not usually go to school, then the teaching staff and play specialists can provide some alternative activities for them to do in their room. For many older children, however, a short session in the school room provides a welcome break from the monotony of hospital routines and endless TV.

Therapists

Families may meet many different (and wonderful) therapists depending on the child's condition.

- *Art, music and play therapists* support a child (and sometimes siblings) to process some of their feelings around their illness, condition or treatment. They use art, music or play as a medium through which to address emotional or psychological issues that the child is finding difficult.
- *Dietitians* are specialists in figuring out a child's nutritional requirements, growth or weight gain and food intake. They may be involved if a child has allergies, food reactions, a complex condition that makes it hard for them to get enough calories, or a physical difficulty with eating. They are also involved with children who are enterally (via nasogastric or gastrostomy tube) or parenterally (intravenously) fed. There's often a fine balance between ensuring the correct calorie and nutritional intake, and protecting the normality of feeding and eating.
- *Occupational therapists* are experts at helping children who struggle to maintain the activities of daily living. This may involve providing therapeutic devices such as splints, wedges, cushions, and other equipment, as well as advising on postural support, exercises, movement and home adaptations. Some OTs will also provide input with various sensory difficulties.

- *Physiotherapists* support children with various conditions or disability if they have a particular movement or musculoskeletal problem. Some physiotherapists also work with children with neurological or neurodevelopmental challenges or respiratory conditions. They usually use a variety of exercises, movements and therapeutic equipment to support improvement in function or range of movement.
- *Speech and language therapists* support children to develop to their full potential in speech, language and communication. They also support children with airway, feeding and swallowing challenges. They may work with a child individually or in a group, on the ward, in an outpatient clinic or at school, depending on their condition and challenge, and like all therapeutic work, parents will be involved in their support and care packages.

On the ward

While a child is resident on the ward, it will probably be very different to home, but most people soon get used to the usual routines and activities. Here is what to expect, and some tips to pass the time for you to share with families, or utilise yourself if you are on the ward with a child you look after.

The daily routine

Hospitals run on routine. As someone known to be an advocate for responsive, child-led parenting, this fact grates a little. But in fairness, hospitals are caring for thousands of sick people, employing hundreds of staff, and managing countless procedures every day. It would probably all fall apart if there was not some predictability and order!

Families will perceive a few regular rhythms to their day:

On the ward

Shift changes

Most of the therapists, administrative and auxiliary staff have an 8-4 or 9-5 working pattern. Clinicians work around the clock in shifts, with the nursing staff having the most variable patterns. Some nurses may work an 'early' shift, which will be approximately 7am-3pm, or a 'late' shift, which may be 2pm-10pm. Other hospitals have a predominant pattern of 'long days', which are 12.5-hour shifts, covering 24 hours. These shifts are usually about 8am-8.30pm or 8pm-8.30am (the night shift). The half hour overlap allows for the nursing shift 'handover', when the nurse in charge of the previous shift will hand over key details of the current inpatients to the new shift.

If you spend any amount of time on the ward at the beginning or end of the day, you will notice an influx of new, fresh faces, but possibly also in the middle of the day as well. This affects families directly, because they will be allocated a nurse who will oversee any clinical care the child needs during their shift. They will hand over care of the child to the next nurse taking over, rather like handing on a baton in a relay race. This ensures that each child's care is continuous.

Ward round

The daily ward round is usually when a child's care and treatment plan are discussed, along with any changes to their condition. It is usually led by the paediatrician and there may be several doctors present, as well as at least the nurse in charge, and possibly the nurse looking after the child that shift. In some hospitals or wards, therapists are also present. It is generally also a chance for the team to talk to parents and find out how their child is getting on. The entire ward round can take a few hours depending on how many patients there are to review and how complex the children's care on the ward or unit is.

When it is an individual child's turn to be seen, the team will usually make plans – which may include new tests, procedures, medication changes, or even plans for discharge home. For this reason, many parents eagerly await the ward round, hoping for news, progress or a plan. It is always a good idea to advocate for a family for whom English is not their first language to have an interpreter present for the ward round. Having a sick child is stressful enough without the additional burden of either having to work harder to translate and decode language, or risk gaps in understanding. If an interpreter is required, it helps to make sure that if the family has any questions, they write them down, so they are not forgotten. It is also sensible to make sure that any other important conversations requiring interpretation take place at the same time – many interpreters are in high demand, and it is not always easy to get them back to the ward as their remit is usually for the whole hospital.

Meals

Although many people complain about hospital food, the regular meals in hospital provide a solid anchor to the day. Breakfast, lunch and dinner (and often snacks and drinks) are served at the same times every day, usually via a trolley or cart that comes into the ward from the ward kitchen. The catering team will make sure everyone gets the meal they ordered, including any special meals. There may be provision for some parents to be provided with food depending on individual hospital policies. Some breastfeeding mothers are provided with food, although my own research found that this was patchy, inconsistent and subject to staff discretion (Hookway et al., 2023). Personally, I genuinely believe that *anyone* who is resident with a sick child in hospital should be provided with food because the alternative is that a child may have to be left alone (unsafe), in the care of busy clinical staff (unrealistic), or with another parent on the ward (inappropriate) while the parent buys food. Often, when food is not provided, parents are encouraged to ask friends or family to bring in food for them, but this is not always possible if a family is isolated or the hospital is far from their home. On-site canteens and shops are also often expensive and there are limited food choices, which increases both the emotional and financial burden. This may be one area where those involved with a family may be able to help – arranging a meal delivery schedule could be invaluable to families on the ward who have limited options and don't particularly want to survive on the contents of vending machines or overpriced packaged sandwiches.

Obs

Clinical observations, or 'obs' for short, are important measurements of a child's physical condition. This includes the child's temperature, pulse, respiration rate, oxygen saturations, blood pressure, capillary refill time, neurological status and pain score. Children may not have all these observations. For example, if they have had an infection, the clinical staff will need to know about signs of infection, so will monitor temperature, pulse and respiratory rate, but their neurological score might be less relevant. If a child has been admitted to hospital the night before a routine minor surgical procedure, they may need even less monitoring than this.

A paediatric early warning (PEW) score is often calculated at the same time as a child's obs. This is a score based on the child's physiological condition, and it helps clinicians to objectively determine whether the child's condition is changing. As a result of an increase in PEW score, children may have more frequent checks, or an earlier review by a doctor, for example. Debate is ongoing about exactly which

PEW score is the most accurate, but most people agree that PEW scores in general can identify deteriorating children and improve multidisciplinary working (Lambert et al., 2017).

A pain score should be calculated if a child is in pain, or they are on medication for pain. Pain scores are more difficult to use in paediatrics, as this is a highly heterogenous group, with different ages, cognitive abilities, conditions, communication skills and levels of pain (Manocha and Taneja, 2016). However, there are scores that can be used for children who are pre-verbal, as well as verbal. Children who can verbally communicate may be asked to rate their pain from 'no pain at all' to 'the worst pain ever' using a scale of smiley/sad faces, or a numeric score from 1–5.

Accurately recorded obs enable clinicians to make decisions about treatment and care based on how each child is responding. The standard obs routine is four-hourly – often 6am, 10am, 2pm, 6pm, 10pm and 2am. However, children whose condition is less stable will have obs recorded more frequently, as their condition warrants, and some children are monitored continuously – for example if they are in intensive care. Other times, they will temporarily be more frequently monitored – such as during a blood transfusion, after a head injury or post-operatively.

Most obs are recorded by nurses, though healthcare assistants and student nurses may also do these, feeding back any concerns to the nurse in charge of the child's care. Many parents become experts in knowing what is typical for their child and can inform their nurse of changes that are worrying to them.

Medications

Most children are likely to receive medication while they are in hospital. These medications may be oral, inhaled, topical, intravenous or injected. How frequently these are given depends on the drug, the child's condition and their treatment plan. Some medications are given just once a day, whereas others are given every 3, 4, 6, 8 or 12 hours. Others are given hourly, and yet more are given 'when required'. Each child will have their own drug chart, and this will list the medications to be given, with a space for them to be signed off once they are administered. Check with your child's nurse about medications you usually give at home. Often these are stored in the medicine room to make sure they are safe, and to ensure there is no accidental double-dosing. You may still be able to give your child their medication. If, for example, the child is more comfortable with *you* (rather than a nurse) giving an inhaler, nebuliser, injection or tablet, it is usually perfectly alright for the nursing staff to bring the medication, and you to administer it. Just check in with the team so everyone knows your preferences, as there may be a competency document that is required to be signed off before someone who is not a member of staff may perform certain tasks.

Differences between weekdays and weekends

One difference to mention is that weekends and weekdays have a distinctly different pace and feel. Many of the staff only work during the week, and (apart from the nursing staff) those that do work weekends may have different working hours. There will still be a ward round, but it will likely be later in the day, and have fewer doctors. Unless it is an emergency, there will be no scans or other tests. There are fewer people buzzing around and generally anything that is routine will wait until Monday. Some families prefer this slower pace, while others find it more frustrating. You will find that come Monday morning, there is a distinct gear shift and a sense of catching up on all the jobs.

Why Childhood Illness Matters

Ward maintenance

Quite apart from the clinical routines, there are all the other activities and tasks that take place on a predictable rhythm as well. The housekeeping staff will swoop in, usually at least once a day, to sweep the floor (handy if a toddler was given a tub of glitter by the play team!) and dust the surfaces. Domestic staff will also empty the bins regularly – it's amazing how quickly they fill up. The child and their parent will be visited by someone who will take the food order for the day. This is all before the routine fire alarm testing, linen delivery trolleys, and the ever-present call of 'has anyone got the keys?' (the keys to the drug cupboard are always in the possession of a registered nurse and obviously, if that nurse is mid-procedure in cubicle 7 at the end of the corridor, it can take some time to track them down).

Noise, lights and sensory overload

I feel it is worth mentioning that hospitals are not just scary places, but loud, bright, and overwhelming places too. Phones ring, bleeps alarm, monitors beep, people yell, laugh, cry, shout and chatter. The lights are (necessarily) bright, there are coloured lights and flashing lights from monitors, torches shine in eyes and throats. There are the smells of disinfectants, people's takeaway food, burned toast, strong perfume, unmentionable smells, and, of course, the combined smell of illness and 50 people in close proximity. There isn't a moment's peace or privacy, and this can leave many parents feeling edgy and stressed, and more so if they are neurodivergent or sensitive to multiple sensory inputs. I wish I had a foolproof way of handling this reality, but the truth is, many of these overwhelming sensory inputs are unavoidable. Here are some strategies to take the edge off:

On the ward

- Loop ear plugs reduce the amount of noise you are exposed to without shutting out sound completely.
- Bone-conducting earphones allow people to zone out with a podcast or music, but do not stop them from hearing background noise.
- Eye masks will help with all the lights overnight.
- Parents can bring a pillow or blanket from home if this helps them feel more comfortable.
- Suggest bringing small comforts like slippers, soft socks, warm scarves or treats such as snacks to cheer them up and calm them down.

I know these small things won't completely stop the ward from being a mind-blowing place for many people, which is why my final tip is that parents try to share the load with someone they trust. A partner, grandparent, relative, or close friend the child knows may offer to relieve them for a while so they can get off the ward and have a break. I'll come back to this in chapters 6 and 8.

Keeping boredom at bay

While it may not be the first thing on most people's minds when they think about having a sick child in hospital, boredom can be a huge problem for both parents and children. In hospital, it is obviously much harder to occupy yourself and a child because there is not the access to usual activities, spaces and people. Here are some tips to manage:

- If the child is old enough and well enough, encourage them to go to school.
- Ask the play specialists for some age-appropriate activities for the child. If you know you will be in hospital over the

weekend, plan ahead and ask for a couple of activities or crafts to do.
- Play games: I-spy, noughts and crosses, guess my animal, hangman and travel board games are good for older children, and for toddlers try colouring, sticker books, simple puzzles and books.
- Unless the child is in protective isolation, see if any friends or family can come and visit – this provides a huge morale boost and change in conversation.
- Maintain connections with home and friends via videocall.
- Do not feel guilty about TV!

What to bring

Finally, many families keep a pre-packed hospital bag in the car, or by the front door, in case of an emergency dash to hospital. For some the distance to hospital is significant, so popping home to grab another shirt or the phone charger is just not practical.

It may be helpful to have a list of recommended items to pack in a hospital bag. Many families in a crisis can't remember what things they will need to bring. It's not patronising to ensure that stressed parents have the items that will be essential for them. One tip is to pack the bag, but then also have a couple of grab bags with changes of clothes for child and parent so that people visiting from home can bring the grab bag and swap it out for dirties when they visit, then launder the clothes and repack the capsule bag. It can be very difficult to manage this on the ward. Not all wards and units have laundry facilities, and with some wards being boiling hot and others being freezing cold, it can be hard to stay comfortable and fresh.

Another good tip is to pack earplugs – as mentioned, hospitals are exceptionally noisy places. Phone chargers,

Kindles and iPads are also useful, though parents should take care of valuable electronics because sadly some unattended possessions do get stolen. Depending on the age of the child, some favourite games might be lifesavers, and for younger children, bringing small activities to while away long and boring hours on the ward is invaluable.

It's also a good idea to pack non-perishable snacks – popcorn, dried fruit, granola bars and sachets of hot chocolate or herbal tea bags to make your favourite hot drink, rather than hospital-issue coffee! I caution parents about valuables but I do recommend a small amount of cash for essential emergency purchases. Some parents can work from hospital, so bringing what they need to get by for a day or two saves a lot of wasted time.

Remember breast pads, sanitary products, a breast pump if needed and contact lens solution – it's inconvenient to be caught without these – and I also suggest you have an emergency supply of painkillers that are in a child-safe bottle. There's nothing worse than having a splitting headache on the paediatric ward – and it's not that easy to get hold of some ibuprofen if you're not the actual patient.

Don't forget things like a notebook to write down questions, and a comfort object for your child if they are attached to a particular toy.

But finally, everyone is human, and things do get forgotten. If you dashed to hospital and forgot everything except the car keys, ask the nurses as they might have some emergency supplies. Failing that, get a family member or friend to bring your essentials in – you could leave grab bags and travel-sized toiletries in an easy-to-find location so that emergency supplies can be delivered.

4
Family-centred care

One of the interventions proposed to mitigate some of the stress of paediatric hospital admission is family-centred care. You might find this hard to believe, but it is a relatively recent development that parents are now encouraged to remain resident with a child overnight. Children used to be admitted to the ward and kept in isolation, with only infrequent visits from their family. Concerns around the impact of this practice began to escalate from about the 1940s (Van der Horst & Van der Veer, 2008). Family-centred care is now the accepted best practice for caring for infants and children in paediatrics, but it wasn't always the case. Progress was only really made following extensive work by various researchers who were exploring attachment.

Attachment is the enduring emotional bond that connects two people across time and space (Ainsworth, 1979). The primary attachment figure and the attachment relationship that a child has will shape their lifelong experiences and chances. Broadly speaking, when a child receives responsive care from their primary attachment figure, they will develop stronger, closer, and more secure bonds with others, as well as optimise brain development. John Bowlby argued in 1969 that in the early months of life a child has distinct and pre-programmed behaviours designed to facilitate parental proximity. This is often referred to as 'dependence' and manifests as a child wanting to be held by their mother, for example, or crying that does not stop until they are picked up.

How children attach

There are many theories of how attachment occurs. Schaeffer and Emerson (1964) proposed four stages of attachment:

1. *0–6 weeks: infants are asocial.* At this age, infants do not purposefully smile at people and faces. Smiles do occur, but they are generally random, and not usually true social smiles in response to social stimuli.
2. *6 weeks–7 months: indiscriminate attachment.* Infants in this age group enjoy social interaction with almost anyone. They do seem to prefer familiar people and can be more quickly comforted by a familiar caregiver, but generally get upset if social interaction is withheld regardless of who is paying them attention.
3. *7–9 months: specific attachment.* At this age, infants show a preference for one person over anyone and everyone else. They are wary of strangers and display distress at being separated from their specific attachment figure. This distress is widely seen as evidence of an attachment to a particular person.
4. *10 months and older: multiple attachments.* As infants get older, they are capable of forming several attachments – for example to another parent, grandparents, a carer, or other responsive adult.

Later, a child's attachment behaviours are driven by conditions that the child can't manage or struggles to cope with – such as pain, discomfort, dysregulation, tiredness, hunger, or distress. Adults display these behaviours as well, but they may be directed toward a partner, trusted family member or friend. For example, if an adult experiences bad news, grief, or they are sick, they may desire close contact with a partner or family member. This is highly relevant of course when we are thinking about sick children, as distressed children and parents alike may exhibit these proximity-seeking behaviours and require more comfort and active calming strategies.

The growth of attachment theory leading to (slow!) hospital policy change

Prior to about 1960, the predominant theory was that infants were incompetent, unable to see, hear or feel at birth, and that their primary motivation to develop a relationship with an adult was through a conditioned response. The theory was that infants form a relationship because they come to associate an adult with the provision of food. John Watson (1913) argued that behaviours were a construct of cause and effect, and reflex actions. He studied children who were growing up in hospital, fed by wet nurses, and observed their learned behaviours, fears, and responses to certain stimuli. He and many other theorists believed that infants primarily stay close to a caregiver because of the provision of food. Children were not thought to have emotional needs, and kissing, holding, hugging, and responding to crying were widely thought of as indulgent and unnecessary behaviours.

Many of the modern attachment theories stem from the seminal work done in the 1940s–80s and draw on earlier work by Freud and Piaget.

Family-centred care

1930: *John Bowlby* was working as a psychiatrist, mostly working with very disturbed children. He began to research the impact of the early environment on the development of the infant.

1947: *Rene Spitz* produced a film, called 'Grief: A Peril in Infancy', which demonstrated (heartbreakingly) the impact of long-term separation of mothers and babies. You can view this film on YouTube but be warned, you may find it distressing.

1958: *Harry Harlow* began his work in non-human primates, demonstrating the importance of love, even over food.

1958: *John Bowlby* began to challenge the widely held view that an infant's primary need is for food – essentially 'cupboard love'.

1959: Publication of the *Platt Report*. This recommended that children should have more access to their parents during hospitalisation. (Full implementation of this report was still not achieved in a survey of UK hospitals in 1988. By as late as 1993, while most hospitals had unrestricted visiting for children in hospital, there was still room for improvement in adolescent care.)

1961: *John Bowlby* published his work on separation anxiety, arguing that infants and young children exhibit a sequence of predictable behaviours when apart from their attachment figure.

1962: *Margaret Ainsworth* began to talk about the effects of maternal deprivation on infants. She later went on to investigate types of attachment in her 'Strange Situation' experiment, which is still used today.

1974: *Thomas Berry Brazelton* started to persuade the wider medical field that infants are competent and able to communicate effectively from birth. His work expanded into the observation of subtle infant cues and attunement and responsiveness to these cues.

1975: *James Prescott* theorised that more carrying, touch and meeting the primary needs of infants – proximity, touch and motion – reduced later violence and aggression. He observed 49 cultures/societies to prove his theory.

1987: *Michael Rutter* published his work on protective mechanisms and psychosocial factors relating to child vulnerability. His ideas (still used in social work and children's public health today) focus on reducing risks, establishing and maintaining self-esteem, and reducing vulnerability by finding opportunities, whether these are other caring and invested adults, school, or childcare.

1994: *Allan Schore* published his work on affect regulation and emotional development. He is particularly interested in the effects of trauma and infant brain development.

You can see that work on attachment is not new, and although it has developed over time, the overarching theme is that small children generally do better when they are promptly responded to, and shown unconditional love, affection, and touch. These were radical ideas until at least the 1980s, and many people needed a lot of convincing that children needed love more than strict discipline.

These early attachment pioneers are largely responsible for why parents now remain resident with their hospitalised children. It has sparked change in social care, hospital policies and daycare recommendations. Prior to this work, if children were unwell and required hospitalisation, they would only be allowed brief visits from their family, including their mother. The Platt report also recommended changes that have led to children being cared for in designated paediatric clinical areas, by paediatric-trained, rather than adult-trained, nurses.

Family-centred care

The birth of family-centred care

Family-centred care (FCC), foundationally, is about protecting a child's mental health by recognising the importance of attachment. It is at the heart of paediatric healthcare delivery, including within the critical care environment (Young et al., 2006), but this is still sometimes hard to achieve. At its heart, FCC recognises the family as the expert and constant in a child's life and demands effective collaboration and information-sharing between professionals and parents in all areas of healthcare. Exactly how this is interpreted, however, remains loose within different countries, healthcare delivery models, and even from hospital to hospital. While most paediatric facilities would say they are paid-up subscribers to an effective model of family-centred care, in practice, because of the lack of a robust set of standards defining what FCC is, the experiences of families on individual paediatric units may differ significantly (Shields, 2015).

There are some common key misunderstandings of FCC which have, over the years, led to suboptimal delivery of the practice. One misunderstanding is that parents are allowed to be present on the ward so that they can take on many of the practical aspects of 'nursing' their child and thus lighten the nursing staff's workload. I have seen this play out a few times in certain attitudes, for example expecting parents to take on the responsibility for round-the-clock tube feeds, or doing a child's obs. Neither of these activities is necessarily 'wrong' for a parent to do, but the devil is in the detail of how the allocation of these tasks is communicated. Rather than a nurse expecting that a parent will do a tube feed, handing the parent the equipment and then bustling off to do something else, true family-centred care is a partnership. The nurse should allocate the time they need to do the feed, approach the child and parent, and negotiate the task. Would the parent prefer to do the feed today? Would they like to watch and learn? Would the child like to participate? Would the parent like to do it but have the nurse remain present to provide guidance or talk to the child? Would the parent like to do certain parts of the process but not all?

You can see that in this way, far from parental involvement saving time, it may take *more* time, so it is certainly not a justification for fewer members of staff or a reduced skill mix with fewer trained nurses. Indeed, collaboration, parental involvement and partnership in care require more staff, more training, more skill and more time.

Parent stressors

There are many practical and logistical problems associated with having a sick child, such as needing to have time off work, adaptations to lifestyle, relationship strain and loneliness and isolation for the parent resident with the hospitalised child. While the resident parent and child are on the ward, they are unable to access their usual sources of companionship, support, activities, entertainment and exercise, and it is often harder or impractical for other siblings to visit, causing parents to make difficult choices about which child they have most contact with (Ivany et al., 2016; Belanger et al., 2017). Some research has also found that the parents of chronically unwell and disabled children are also themselves more likely to experience poor health (Vonneilich et al., 2016), possibly due to chronic stress, and exacerbated by delaying seeking personal support and care due to prioritising caring for their child.

It is common for parents to struggle with finances and income, and this affects those with lower incomes disproportionately (Beck et al., 2017). While admitted to a ward or PICU, parents often have to purchase food for themselves or their child, and the on-site hospital shopping facilities are usually more expensive (Thomson et al., 2016). Some parents may need to give up paid employment to care for their child (Kish et al., 2018), while others must make adaptations or rely on understanding employers – which adds to their stress. On top of this, parents may have to pay for transport, parking, travel for other family members and associated costs of being away from home. It is hard to maintain usual duties such as laundry, housework and caring for other children while resident on the ward. Juggling work, wider family members, a partner, the home and pets is difficult and stressful, and has an indirect effect on parental mental health and coping ability (van Oers et al., 2014).

What family-centred practices you should expect

Practices vary from hospital to hospital, so you might have a different experience. The following reflects my own interpretation of practical family-centred care and observations of practice over the years. I have chosen to implement family-centred and attachment theory as follows:

Information-sharing

This means that there will often be a set of shared care records, particularly in the case of children with chronic or complex care. A simple example of family-centred information sharing is the personal child health record (known as the 'red book'). This is slowly being digitalised and may also have specialist charts and information for certain conditions. While this is not always filled in by every professional who sees a child, the idea is for this to be a place where information can be seen by everyone. Information-sharing also applies to keeping families in the loop, using clear communication, and being honest about when things go wrong. An accurate history should be taken that accounts for the ideas, concerns, and expectations of the family. Families should know what the working diagnosis and differential diagnoses are, what tests might be needed, the expected duration of treatment and any parts of the child's case that they are not clear about. I believe that information-sharing also encompasses the nursing and medical handover – the information that is pertinent to enable compassionate care of families is not just clinical, but also related to the child and family's preferences and needs.

Respecting and honouring differences
This part of FCC acknowledges that the ward or PICU is a scary and strange place for families and not part of the normal experience of parenting and family life. The ward may be familiar and non-threatening to staff, but it is the opposite for many families. However, despite the environment being alien to families, their knowledge of their child is unparalleled. Valuing parents' knowledge of their child, and their unique insights into a child's response to illness, is key. Honouring differences also means that differences in culture, family values and parenting philosophy should be respected and upheld. In practice, I believe this applies to parenting behaviours, individual arrangements for sleep and responsiveness, feeding, play and social needs, as well as religious, dietary, and cultural preferences and appropriate use of interpreter services as required.

Partnerships and collaboration
This means that the expertise in managing the child should be considered to be equally shared between the clinicians and parents. The parents have expert knowledge of their child, and the clinicians have expert knowledge of the illness and managing sick children. There should be no hierarchy

Family-centred care

of power here, because effective care and treatment of the child requires knowledge of both elements. It also applies to the practical care of the child, which should be sensitively managed. How can the parents be involved? How can families and clinicians help each other? How do they listen to each other respectfully? How does their respective knowledge inform the care of the child? Practically, it also suggests that parents should always be present during the ward round and any discussions about the care and management of the child.

Negotiation

This is perhaps the aspect of FCC that is most open to interpretation! Many aspects of care can be negotiated, from who does what, to when they do it, how often and where. Visiting and involvement can be negotiated. But above all, I believe nuanced conversations with families are a key feature of this aspect of FCC. By that I mean a kind of negotiation of expertise – the family stating what they know and what further information they need to know, and the clinician filling in the gaps as required. So often, clinicians have a spiel and want to say their piece, but true negotiated care would understand that not all families need the same information in the same way. In my experience, it takes a great deal of humility and experience for a clinician to feel comfortable with this type of interaction.

Care in the context of the family and community

This means that all care should account for the needs of the family. The needs of the parents and siblings should feature in decision-making and planning. How the family is coping as a unit should be an important factor in care delivery. The family should be offered the chance to be acquainted with the ward, routines, and staff to reduce anxiety. Food should be provided for those caring for the child on the ward, and facilities that make the family's life easier should be made available, such as laundry, beds, privacy, financial aid, activities, and the freedom to have visitors.

I'm not suggesting that any of this is easy or readily achievable, but if we don't have a lofty goal in mind, there's less progress to aim for! Many units are already excelling, I should stress, and there are many committed paediatric clinicians who live by this philosophy every day. I've been honoured to meet many of them.

What family-centred care could/should look like

For parents to truly be valued as partners in care, and to provide the kind of FCC that makes a difference to the experience of families, we need to consider:

- Sleeping arrangements. I would love to see a full-size parent bed available next to each child's bed, and more nuanced policies around bedsharing and night-time comforting (more on this in Chapter 7). Presently, many parents sleep on reclining chairs or narrow pull-out beds.
- Considering the needs and comfort of parents. This is much more subtle to define, but in an ideal world, with a good working model of FCC, staffing should acknowledge the additional workload of having at least double the number of people to care for. There is always a child and a someone. That someone has needs too. The someone is also in a scary, difficult, stressful place and requires additional support. It isn't fair on nursing staff to expect them to provide this and have no time to practically deliver this kind of care.
- Age-appropriate differentiation of care. Paediatric wards cater for children from birth to at least 16, and this represents a vast range of needs. The needs of a parent

Family-centred care

and newborn are quite obviously different from the needs of a parent and toddler, or school-age child, or teenager. Communication, activities, partnership in care, and allocation of responsibilities need to reflect this.

- Practical needs of families. Children and families do not stop having real-life problems just because of illness. It has always frustrated me how difficult it is to survive on a paediatric ward for any length of time. Parents are completely at the mercy of whatever facilities are available. They have few freedoms or abilities to meet their needs. This includes being able to shop for healthy, nutritious food, wash dirty clothes, have access to play, exercise and education, and access to washing facilities with adequate privacy. Provision of these opportunities would reduce stress.
- Using person-first language and remembering names. Never, ever refer to a child by their illness or diagnosis. It is awful to hear of children being referred to as 'the cystic fibrosis kid' or the 'diabetic girl'. In a similar vein, I have a bee in my bonnet about not calling parents 'mum' or 'dad' (and I'm not the only one). It means the world to be called by your name and not by an impersonal and generic term (Nimmo, 2019). It is also never appropriate to change a parent or child's name to something that is 'easier to say'.
- Emotional, psychological, social, and spiritual needs. Hospitalisation and long-term illness is exhausting, confusing, stressful, and upsetting. Families need to be able to observe cultural and religious practices that are important to them. Parents and children also need adequate opportunities to alleviate some of this stress through psychological support, opportunities for companionship and distraction. While in hospital, most parents and children do not have the opportunity to exercise, and

experience boredom, loneliness, and subsequent effects on their morale.

- Financial support. Unquestionably, having a sick child is expensive, both directly, through the costs of parking, travel, food, and entertainment (emergency online impulse purchases at 3am...) and indirectly, through having to modify employment or give up work entirely. Providing assistance with parking charges, travel and food subsidies would help considerably.

If you are involved in caring for a family who are going through childhood illness, understanding some of these stressors and logistical problems may help you to firstly understand what kind of pressure they are under, and secondly, what support they might find helpful to reduce their stress.

Family-centred critical care

Some studies have found that parents do not feel as involved as they would like when their child is in a critical care environment (Ames et al., 2011; Butler et al., 2014; Hill et al., 2019). There are also additional pressures relating to parenting in a very public environment – especially when a child is in intensive care, where the clinical environment affords little privacy for tender connection, silliness, or expressions of raw vulnerability (Rempel et al., 2013). Some of the common difficulties are around not being able to be present overnight on the paediatric intensive care unit (PICU) with their child, a lack of acceptance of skin-to-skin and nurturing care on PICU, and how traumatic the environment itself was. A recent European survey of PICUs found that only 50% have rooming-in facilities (Nielsen et al., 2022). On one level, this is understandable. If you picture the average intensive care unit, many wards are very open – this is so that all patients can be easily monitored and there is no delay in rapidly accessing a patient who needs immediate care. Many hospitals were designed decades before we all realised that FCC was a good idea, and therefore the existing infrastructure of the ward does not always lend itself to the provision of privacy, or even enough space for a parent bed to be safely placed next to the child, without any resulting negative impact on safety.

But on the other hand, how is it that we still accept parent-child separation as standard during illness, especially critical illness? Many parents describe not being able to be with their child overnight as extraordinarily stressful. If we think about attachment theory again, this is not surprising. We are hard-wired to need to be with our children, and this may be accentuated when they are very unwell. While it may seem kind to encourage parents to get off the stressful PICU and sleep at home, or in hospital accommodation away from the unit's bleeps and buzzes, almost every parent I have ever spoken to has reported poor sleep and more stress despite the opportunity for uninterrupted rest.

Newer models of family-integrated care (FIC) as opposed to family-centred care (FCC) are being successfully adopted in many neonatal units and seem to have a much greater emphasis on keeping the whole family together (van den Hoogen and Ketelaar, 2022) but this has yet to be adopted in paediatrics. We certainly have a long way to go.

What challenges remain and how you can help

There may be many challenges with supporting FCC in paediatrics, but progress is always being made. Those outside healthcare systems may not always fully understand the unique pressures that exist. Perhaps the changes that should be made look obvious. The reality is that change takes time – as evidenced by the amount of time that it took for attachment theory to filter down into hospital policies, and then for that to be implemented in practice. Healthcare evolution can and does happen, but some barriers to change are bigger than others, including physical infrastructure, finances, and staffing.

The good news is that you can help. Family-centred care isn't just for hospitals. You can take and use this information to help you support the families you care for as well. Principles of negotiating care and responsibilities, making time to acknowledge the work of caring for parents as well as children, valuing the role the family has in the life of the child, and trying to minimise the stressors that families experience, will all go a long way.

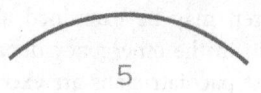

5

Treatments and procedures

Part of the process of illness diagnosis, assessment and management involves tests, treatments and procedures. Not fun, but necessary and understandable. Of course, adults are usually able to have a test explained. Having the risks and benefits, pros and cons, and rationale articulated to us enables us to make an informed choice. For many infants and children, the heavy weight of responsibility for making these decisions lies with their parent, who must also support them through various procedures.

Understanding what the common tests and procedures are can help you to both prepare and support parents and children, and empathise with them when they are discussing or planning for this experience.

Examinations

Although an examination is usually not painful, it can be very intimidating for a young child to be examined. There is a certain vulnerability that is inherent in being physically examined. Children may be examined at the GP surgery, minor injury unit, in the emergency department, clinics or on the ward. Most paediatricians are exceptionally sensitive and child-centred in their approach to examination, but nonetheless it is sometimes intimidating for little ones. Obviously the type and extent of the examination will be determined by what the presenting complaint is. There is no need for a whole-body examination if the child's only complaint is an ingrown toenail. But equally, if the child has a problem with a more intimate part of their body, there is no way of getting around the need to examine that body part. Many children who are inpatients will be examined daily – a child with a skin infection will obviously have their infection looked at to determine the next course of action. A child with sepsis of unknown origin will be examined to try to identify an obvious source of infection, and so on. Even when there is nothing obvious to see, many children will have their chest listened to, or their lymph nodes palpated. Consent and assent are a vital part of examination and it is a doctor's job to ascertain a child's competence to consent, and even in the absence of age and cognitive ability to consent, the child's privacy and dignity should be maintained (De Lourdes et al., 2003). This may involve using a private space, screen, sheet or towel. It may also involve the clinician using compassionate gestures such as warming their hands, using humour, or talking to the child to reassure them. While most examinations are painless, if the child is acutely sore, by definition, touching the part that is sore may be painful. Even if it isn't, there is a discomfort in being examined that should be acknowledged, even though it may be unavoidable, and clinicians will never examine a child unless they have to.

Treatments and procedures

Medications

Another pretty obvious intervention is medication. Some routes of administration are more painful than others. Some are more embarrassing than others. And some are not painful but they are a little scary for small children. Some medications are given via a certain route because of the way in which they are absorbed or metabolised. It is impossible to cover all the reasons a child may need a medication, so I will focus instead on the most common routes in children and how to help them through being given a necessary medication.

Enteral (into the gastrointestinal tract)

- *Oral:* medications that can be given via a syrup, tablet, capsule, suspension, or chewable tablet. This route obviously requires the child to be conscious, have a safe swallow and requires a degree of cooperation to avoid the medicine being spat out or aspirated. Most medicines given at home, such as pain relief or antibiotics, are given orally, or via a child's nasogastric, orogastric, nasojejunal or gastrostomy tube.
- *Buccal:* this is given into the little space between the inner lining of the cheek and gums. This may be used when a child is not conscious, very sleepy or when the drug needs to rapidly take effect. Some medications given in emergencies use this route – for example anti-seizure medication or glucose for hypoglycaemia. The buccal route is also used for mouth care and to provide immune therapy with expressed breastmilk, for example.
- *Rectal:* some medications are given into the rectum via a bullet-shaped suppository. Medications given via this route are often absorbed more quickly and therefore act faster, avoid the need for a safe swallow and cannot be vomited or spat.

Inhaled

- *Inhaler:* a metered-dose inhaler delivers a measured dose of a drug usually in powdered form into the lungs. It requires proper technique to achieve good effect though, so many children who use inhalers use them with a spacer, which is a large plastic chamber that allows you or your child to dispense the inhaler into the spacer and breathe in and out without having to coordinate pressing the inhaler and inhaling at exactly the right time.
- *Nasal:* this is usually a liquid spray or drops. You may yourself have administered a nasal spray for hayfever, sinusitis or even migraine. If you have, you'll know that these drugs can work extremely quickly, but the downside is that they can give a very unpleasant taste in the back of the mouth.
- *Nebuliser:* this is where a small volume of a solution in a chamber is mixed with oxygen to deliver the medication via a mouthpiece into the lungs in tiny droplets. It is commonly used in asthmatic patients as well as those in acute respiratory distress. One of the downsides of this route is that although it is painless, it is noisy as the oxygen creating the aerosol with the liquid makes a hissing sound and creates a smoke-like appearance. Nurses often try to persuade children that it is 'dragon's smoke' or similar, but even so, some children take some time to get used to this and may panic.

Injected

- *Intravenous:* this is a commonly used route for many medications including analgesia, antibiotics, anaesthesia and many more. The child does not have to be conscious, because the medication is given through a cannula into a vein.

Treatments and procedures

- *Intramuscular:* this is a drug given via injection into a large muscle – such as the deltoid or gluteus muscle. Most vaccinations are given via the intramuscular route.
- *Subcutaneous:* similar to the intramuscular route in that this is given via injection, but into the subcutaneous tissue. Some patients administer these drugs themselves – such as heparin or insulin.

Ocular

- This is a medication in ointment or drop form that is administered into the eye. While not necessarily painful, drops can feel uncomfortable or sting a little, depending on the drug, and it can be disconcerting, as everyone's instinct when something comes towards their eye is to blink, so this requires some cooperation.

Otic

- This means a drug that is given in the ear, usually in drop form, to treat a local problem in the ear canal. This usually does not hurt, but the child may need to lie on their opposite side to administer the drops effectively, and stay there for a few moments to avoid most of the liquid coming straight out again!

Skin

- *Topical:* many medications are given in cream, gel, ointment, or shampoo form to be applied straight to the skin. These almost never hurt, but the compliance with applying creams to the skin regularly can directly affect how effective they are. For example, treating eczema can be difficult because applying the creams as often as prescribed is time-consuming and makes a child slippery or greasy,

which may reduce the number of times the treatment is applied. Good education with creams is therefore essential.
- *Transdermal:* some medications are absorbed through the skin via a patch that is usually stuck down. Some anti-emetic (anti-nausea) as well as analgesic medications are applied this way and have the advantage of being painless.

Making the medicine go down

A major concern for many parents is how to persuade children to take medicines that they've been prescribed. With the best will in the world, not all of them can be made to taste palatable. Some are bitter, some are apparently 'banana' or 'strawberry' flavour, but we all know that this is a bit of a stretch! You may have heard of lots of different ways to try to get the medicine down, but what are the pros and cons?

Strategy	Advantages	Disadvantages
Role play with teddy	Can reduce anxiety of the unknown Can be more empowering Child is in control	Not suitable for infants or very young toddlers May have high compliance until the child *actually* tastes it
Use a syringe to squirt it in rapidly rather than on a spoon	Can bypass many of the tastebuds on the tongue Quick	Risk of aspiration if squirted forcefully or centrally Requires mature ability to swallow
Alternate medicine with something pleasant tasting	Can give the child brief breaks which may increase their tolerance for the unpleasant taste	Can be very slow and drag out the process

Treatments and procedures

Mix with fairly strong squash or juice	Can disguise the flavour and therefore increase likelihood that it will be successfully administered	If the child does not finish the juice you have no way of knowing how much medicine they ingested
Put chocolate sprinkles on top of the medicine on a spoon	Novelty factor may improve compliance	High-sugar strategy. May not disguise the flavour
Get them to pinch their nose while they swallow it	Taste is affected by the sense of smell so pinching the nose may reduce the ability of the child to detect the unpleasant flavour	Requires understanding and compliance because an adult should *never* pinch a child's nose for them
Mix with yogurt/ice cream/custard	Can disguise the flavour more successfully than squash or juice. This works particularly well for granules	Same problem as with juice regarding incomplete and unknown dosage so use the smallest amount possible
Wrap the tablets in bread and swallow whole	Completely removes the bitter/chalky aftertaste of a tablet and bread feels like a familiar substance to swallow	Requires a child to be able to swallow a lump. However, I used this with my 3-year-old successfully when she hated the taste of the syrup version.

Sometimes a medication can be given in another form. For example, it may be available as a suspension instead of a tablet. Some (but not all) tablets can be crushed. Some can be given rectally instead of orally. Sometimes there is a similar medication that tastes better or needs to be given less frequently. It's worth checking with the doctor and a pharmacist to see if there are any workarounds to improve compliance.

Procedures

There are many procedures that children may need to undergo either in hospital, clinic or at home. While there may not always be an easy way around this, there are certainly things we can do to make some procedures easier for little ones. By the way – it should hopefully be obvious, but painful procedures should never take place in the child's bed space or cubicle, or in the playroom: these spaces should be safe and free from the association of unpleasant procedures unless it is an emergency.

Blood tests

Blood tests may be required for many different reasons and there are lots of ways of doing it. A nurse, HCA, phlebotomist, or doctor can use a lancet (finger-pricking device) to collect a very small amount of blood. This is not suitable for all blood tests, or those requiring larger volumes. However, if they just want a full blood count, for example, this may work well. Blood can also be taken with a small needle that is immediately removed after the blood has been taken. A skin-numbing cream may be used, and this can be very effective at reducing pain. If a child is going to be given intravenous fluid or medication, the doctors will usually try to get the blood at the same time. They will cannulate first, take the blood, then flush the line and leave the cannula in situ. It is not always possible to use the cannula to take blood subsequently though, so this is often only a strategy that can be utilised before any medications or fluids are going to be given through the line. Finally, if a child has a central line, such as a Hickman line or Port-a-cath, blood can be taken from these lines, which on the plus side is painless for the child (unless their port needs accessing), but on the flip side, accessing a central line obviously requires a nurse who has had further training and can complete the procedure using aseptic non-touch technique, as there is a higher risk of infection and contamination.

Cannulation

To administer intravenous fluid or medication, a child will need a cannula. As with blood tests, an anaesthetic cream or cold spray may be used before the procedure. The cannula is inserted with a needle which is used to position a very thin, flexible, plastic tube into a vein. The needle is then removed, leaving the cannula, which is relatively comfortable to have in situ. The opening to the cannula will have a bung placed on the end and the whole thing will be taped down securely so it is hard for it to fall out. In very young infants and children they may also use a splint and bandage as well – this is mostly to protect the cannula when children play and crawl around. Sadly, cannulas do not last forever, especially if they are in a thin or precarious vein, so if a child needs intravenous medication or fluid for more than 3–5 days, they may need a fresh cannula.

Positioning children for blood tests and cannulas

Unless it is a medical emergency, the clinical staff will always try to minimise pain and distress with:

- Good pain relief
- Good positioning and holding
- Distraction and play therapy

Pain relief. The person who will take the blood or site the cannula will first have a look at the child's hands, arms, legs, and feet. Occasionally a scalp vein may be used, but this is not the first choice. The clinician will assess which sites are the most likely to be successful, and then, provided there is time, numbing cream will be applied to all the areas. This is because there is nothing more frustrating than finding that the best-looking site to cannulate is the only place that has not had numbing cream! The cream will be allowed to stay on the skin for enough time for it to work (usually 30–60 minutes depending on the brand). Cold spray is often used if there is no time to use cream.

Good positioning and holding. Once the cream has had time to work, usually the most successful position is known as the 'cuddle hold'. The parent sits on a chair, and their child sits on their lap, chest to chest, effectively hugging their parent or carer. The clinician will then crouch or sit to take the blood or site the cannula.

Distraction and play therapy. While the clinician is looking and working, this is where the play team work their magic. Cannulating and taking blood can be painless (honestly!) if cream is used and the child remains unafraid and still. Looking at what the clinician is doing usually causes stress, so the play team are wizards at selecting toys, gadgets, or activities to distract the child. Bubbles and sound and light toys are favourites with very young children. Sometimes TV or talking to the child is the best way.

Treatments and procedures

You can see it's quite a team effort, and paediatric staff really do try their hardest to not cause stress and trauma.

Lumbar puncture

Lumbar punctures are where a small sample of cerebrospinal fluid is taken from the back. A needle is inserted between two vertebrae and the fluid is collected into a sample bottle and sent to the laboratory to test for red and white blood cells, protein, glucose, and bacteria. It is done to diagnose infections of the brain and spinal cord including meningitis, some autoimmune conditions, and some cancers. Numbing cream unfortunately does not work well for this procedure, and one of the keys to success is getting the child in a good position, which involves them being in a curl with their knees near their chin to allow space between the vertebrae to collect the sample. Children with cancer who sometimes need regular lumbar punctures will have this procedure done under a general anaesthetic to minimise their distress. However, a lumbar puncture is more commonly performed to try to diagnose illness in an acutely unwell child with sepsis, and in this case it is not practical or safe to wait to be able to do it under anaesthesia.

Other tests

There are many other tests that may be necessary, from the painless but time-consuming and tricky urine samples, to the waiting game of a stool sample! There are also various scans that a child may need.

Ultrasound scan. This involves a child having some gel placed over the area that needs to be scanned, and the radiographer using a probe to gently press on the anatomy that needs investigation to generate an image. A radiologist will then interpret this image to guide clinical decision-making. The gel is often placed in a warmer, but occasionally it can be cold, which may be unpleasant for some children.

ECG. An electrocardiogram measures electric activity in the heart with sticky sensors placed on a child's chest. The sensors record the activity of the heart and generate a paper or digital representation of what the heart is doing. A child will need to undo or loosen their top, which can be awkward for girls who are self-conscious about their developing breasts, so a loose cropped top which they don't mind getting gel on can help.

CT or MRI scan. Computed Tomography (CT) scans use X-rays and Magnetic Resonance Imaging (MRI) scans use radio waves to look at and provide images of tissues, organs, and bones. They both involve lying down on a bed inside a large scanner. The hardest part about these scans is that the child needs to be quite still. For young infants, the 'feed and wrap' technique is often used, whereby a child is fed until they fall asleep and then they're wrapped comfortably and everyone hopes they sleep through the scan! For older children, the play specialists are often able to explain the procedure using puppets, role play and other techniques to help children tolerate the procedure, which although painless, may be scary and loud. As a last resort, some children have a scan under sedation or general anaesthetic.

X-ray. This is used to produce images, particularly of skeletal structures, but also to look for foreign objects (either accidental – like swallowed coins or objects, or intentional – like the position of a central line or nasojejunal tube). They can also be used to look at some soft structures or identify free air or fluid – for example the lungs, heart, and certain organs. X-rays also require a child to be still, which can be difficult.

Treatments and procedures

One option is for a parent (who is not pregnant) to wear a lead apron and hold their child. The radiographers are also really good at using positioning aids to get good images.

Being with a child for a procedure

While hospitals may have individual rules and regulations about whether parents or carers can be in the room with the child while they have a procedure, it is becoming more and more accepted that this is best practice. Parental presence seems to reduce pain (Azak et al., 2022) and may also reduce stress (Matziou et al., 2013). Although this may seem surprising, parental presence even during resuscitation is also sometimes welcomed (Dainty et al., 2021).

So what might be the arguments for *not* having a parent present during a procedure? There are three main reasons cited in the academic literature:

1. It may negatively impact the performance of the healthcare team (essentially, it is off-putting and nerve-wracking to have parents watch clinically difficult procedures that require skill) (Compton et al., 2006). This can be exacerbated when there is a trainee performing the procedure. As I have previously mentioned, everyone needs to train somehow and at some point, *everyone* needs to do their first 'real person' lumbar puncture, cannula, catheter, or nasogastric tube insertion.
2. There is often a fear of litigation if family members are present, especially during resuscitation (Jensen and Kosowan, 2011). On the other hand, some suggest that litigation is reduced when parents are present as they can *see* what happened (McClenathan et al., 2002).
3. Insufficient staff to be able to support family members during invasive procedures or resuscitation (Sak-Dankosky

et al., 2014). Quite reasonably, some clinical staff point out that there are two needs in this moment – one is to perform the procedure effectively, safely, and competently, and the other is to provide the necessary emotional support at a distressing time to family members. If there are not enough staff present, the worst-case scenario is that the clinician is not able to perform their task, or the parent is left unsupported and in great distress.

Anecdotally, I have had many parents tell me that they were told that it would be too stressful for them to be present, and they have had to wait outside the procedure room, unable to offer their child comfort. All of them have told me that even though they wouldn't have been able to change the fact that their child needed a painful or upsetting procedure, they felt tremendous guilt that they were not there to support them. It is often worse to regret *not* doing something than to regret doing it. While you may not have much influence over individual hospital policies, you may be able to support families as they make decisions about when and how to be present during procedures.

Surgery

If children need to have surgery – either as a planned or emergency procedure – this can be a nerve-wracking experience for families. There are several aspects of surgery that might feel stressful, whether it is a child's first surgical procedure, or their fifteenth.

Consent and pre-op assessments

The first part of the process is that the parent will consent to the surgery. A member of the anaesthetic team will visit the child and parent on the ward and obtain consent for the anaesthesia. They will work out the best way to anaesthetise the child and make sure the child is fit and stable enough for anaesthesia.

Fasting for surgery and how to cope

The next thing to contend with is keeping a child away from food and certain fluids before their surgery. Different hospitals have slightly different policies, but a recent European review (Frykholm et al., 2022) of anaesthetic guidelines summarised the existing evidence and found:

Substance	Fasting time prior to anaesthesia
Clear fluids/water	1 hour
Breastmilk (including fortified breastmilk)	3 hours
Cow's milk (including formula milk)	4 hours
Light breakfast (such as cereal with milk)	4 hours
Solid food (all other solids)	6 hours

These updated recommendations do not differ for children who were born preterm, have reflux, a history of cardiac disease, repaired oesophageal atresia, type 1 diabetes, children who are obese, or those who are nasogastric or gastrostomy tube-fed. However, it is still more common practice to maintain a four-hour fasting policy for all children (ABM, 2012).

Of course, anyone who has held a child who wants to feed or eat and may not, knows that it is extremely hard to cope with. Children usually tolerate fasting until approximately the time that they would usually eat, or are reminded of food, and then all bets are off. Carrying younger children in a sling can help. Distraction and play are also good – although you'll just have to hope nobody is eating in the playroom! Remember that just because a child needs to fast, there is no sense in the parent or carer being hungry or thirsty too. Obviously it would be insensitive to eat in front of the child, but one tip to suggest to parents is that they try to sneak off away from their child and quickly eat. They cannot easily take care of a child who is hungry and irritable if their own basic needs are not met.

Anaesthetics

When it is time for the child to go to surgery, the parent or carer will usually be invited into the anaesthetic room, which is usually a small room just off the operating theatre. Paediatric anaesthetic rooms are much more child-friendly and the staff often go to great lengths to alleviate child and parental anxiety. The nurse caring for the child that shift will accompany them to the anaesthetic room and from there, the anaesthetist and nurses will prepare the child for either their intravenous induction of anaesthesia, or gas induction. There may be compelling clinical reasons to induce anaesthesia in one or other of these ways, which will have been discussed with the family earlier. The child is often allowed to watch a movie or TV show, or sometimes someone will blow bubbles or play with the child to calm them. Parents may hold their child's hand, sit with them, or stroke them as they fall asleep. Once asleep, the parent will be promptly escorted out by the accompanying ward nurse so that the clinical team can intubate the child and then get on with the surgery/procedure.

Passing the time

Many parents find the time while their child is in surgery very stressful.

> '*When my kids had MRIs or surgeries I would always take a walk first when they had to leave my side. I would always bring something to do but allow myself to choose not to do that thing and just sit after my walk if I needed to.*' Brittney Piper

Whether parents walk, read, crochet, call a friend or pace the floor is probably highly personal and they might not have the same response every time even if they are veterans of paediatric surgery – after all, no two surgical procedures are the same, and sometimes the stakes are higher, or the context is different. But empathising with what parents are enduring is a good place to start.

Recovering from surgery

Once a child has had their procedure, their anaesthetic will be stopped. Because these drugs are fast-acting, and quickly eliminated by the body, most people regain consciousness very quickly after the anaesthetist stops actively managing their anaesthesia, and they are moved to the recovery area. Once they have been extubated and are physiologically stable, the ward will be called and the parent may go to be with their child while they wake up properly. As soon as the child is ready, they will then return to the ward. Some children wake up easily from anaesthetic, while others are irritable and cry or shout. Others simply want to sleep. Depending on what procedure the child has had, they will usually have had some analgesia, but the parent will be given instructions on any wounds, stitches, medications, or anything else they need to know.

Pain

Nobody likes to think of their child being in pain, but the reality is that some illnesses, and treatments for illnesses and conditions, sometimes bring pain. Exactly how pain is managed depends on the child's condition, as well as their age and many other individual factors. Pain relief is either pharmacological or non-pharmacological.

Pharmacological: this involves giving a child medication for their pain – either orally, intravenously, intramuscularly, transdermally or whatever is most clinically appropriate. Many paediatric teams will use a pain ladder and a multi-modal approach to pain relief to ensure safe and effective analgesia (Yaster, 2010). Often smaller doses are given to start, and combinations of non-steroidal and steroidal medicines along with non-pharmacological approaches to try to achieve good comfort levels. A pain assessment should also be used alongside pain relief, with reassessment to ensure that the child's pain is under control (Vittinghoff et al., 2018).

Non-pharmacological: there are many approaches to non-pharmacological pain relief, including distraction, play, guided relaxation, massage, and acupuncture (Yaster, 2010). Breastfeeding is known to be an effective form of pain relief for infants and young children, and in large studies has been found to be effective for managing vaccination and heel-stick pain, though I have found in my wider research that many mothers report good pain relief for more significant pain (Shah et al., 2012; Harrison et al., 2016; Harrison and Bueno, 2023). For children who are not breastfed, sucrose water has been shown to be effective (Stevens et al., 2016). There is no research exploring the use of skin-to-skin contact for children beyond the neonatal period, but there is no physiological reason why children should not be held and comforted as much as possible, since the research on skin-to-skin for physiological stability and pain relief is unequivocal (Johnston et al., 2017).

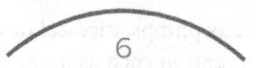

Caring for children with complex illnesses, conditions and disabilities

Some illnesses and conditions are lifelong, and many parents will have to learn how to care for their child with complex needs. You may be involved with children who have complex needs in several ways, and a key point with these families is that they are often experts by experience. I have met countless inspirational parents who walk the difficult line between being their child's parent and their nurse or carer.

Parents of children with complex needs may have to deal with:

- Shock, trauma, and fatigue
- Relapse and remission of their condition
- Recurrent hospitalisation
- Coordinating multiple appointments, with multiple different professionals and services
- Surgery, tests, and procedures
- Home care
- Multiple medications, home oxygen or tube feeding

- Equipment such as pumps, medical devices, and intensive or invasive intervention such as home ventilation or other respiratory support
- Hospices and respite

While every family is different, and the specific healthcare needs of children are unique, there are some common stressors and challenges.

Caring for families of children with complex medical needs at home

More and more children are living with chronic illness or medical complexity, and much of this care takes place at home, although some evidence suggests that children experience ongoing and recurrent health crises which generally worsen over time (Namachivayam et al., 2010). Parents of medically complex children become experts not only on their child, and their child's condition, but also on *exactly* how to manage their child's condition and the way *their* child responds to their condition. In essence, they become hyper-specialised in looking after one patient with a specific condition. But this expertise and specialism can be a confusing experience to navigate alongside the broader knowledge and experience of healthcare professionals, as well as negotiating care and decision-making (Rennick et al., 2019).

The expertise of parents also comes at a psychological cost. Many studies have explored the experience of diagnosis, including the development of post-traumatic stress disorder (Woolf et al., 2016). There are also other negative psychological impacts, including stress, trauma (Pinquart, 2019), anxiety and decreased quality of life (Fairfax et al., 2019), and isolation during PICU admission (Wright-Sexton et al., 2020). Some researchers have differentiated between classic post-traumatic stress disorder and paediatric medical traumatic stress (PMTS), which is positioned as an ongoing and evolving psychological and physiological response to illness, pain, injury, procedures, and experiences (Kazak et al., 2005).

But of course, if you speak to most parents of children with chronic illness, disability, or care needs, they will also speak of the positives: joy, privilege, courage, resilience, hope, connectedness, meaning, self-efficacy and more. Ultimately, most parents, while acknowledging the hard work, would simultaneously tell you that they care for their child fundamentally because they love them. They do not want to be thought of as selfless, heroic or as superheroes – they are simply parents doing their best for their child.

However, there is no doubt that caring for a child with complex needs brings huge responsibility, has significant impacts on daily life and brings a necessary medical element to a family's daily routine. It may also affect relationships and social life and some studies have found an increased risk of poorer mental and physical health among the parents of chronically unwell children (Cohn et al., 2020; Feudtner et al., 2021). Financial stressors are caused by needing to give up paid work, needing to self-fund products, equipment and support, and emergency purchases simply to survive another hospital admission, or pay for parking, travel, and food. There may be financial support available, so it's always worth talking to the hospital social worker to establish whether the family are eligible for any other assistance.

Clinical care in the home

Many children with medical complexity have sophisticated healthcare needs at home including ventilation, tracheostomy, enteral or parenteral feeding and central lines. Parents can become experts in managing these devices and clinical caregiving procedures, which may include:

Respiratory support

Some children require oxygen therapy at home – which may be administered through nasal cannula or mask, and continuously or just overnight depending on their condition. While it is impossible to cover all the reasons a child may need some form of respiratory support, there are some common scenarios. Generally, a child will be prescribed supplemental oxygen, continuous positive airway pressure via a non-invasive face mask, or ventilation via a tracheostomy. Common reasons for home respiratory support include developmental disability, craniofacial anomaly, severe obesity, sleep apnoea, and neuromuscular disease (Järvelä et al., 2023).

One reason for home oxygen is bronchopulmonary dysplasia (chronic lung disease) following a history of premature birth. If a child is stable enough to be cared for at home, but is still oxygen dependent, it may be deemed appropriate for the child to go home on supplemental oxygen. This means that oxygen will be supplied to the home, and the family will also be given smaller oxygen cylinders so that they can still get out and about. You may well have seen small babies with an oxygen cylinder in the bottom of their pushchair. These infants will still be under the care of the neonatal team and will be visited by the neonatal outreach nurses who will monitor their condition, and assess their readiness to be weaned off the oxygen. The support to be weaned off oxygen does vary by area, and depends on the skill mix and home equipment available. You can easily imagine that many parents find home oxygen stressful and equally there are risks of over-oxygenating children, so it is important that they are weaned off the oxygen when it is safe to do so.

Once a child's growth and feeding are satisfactory and there are no concerns about developmental outcomes, they may be suitable for an overnight oxygen saturation study to monitor oxygen saturations during sleep so that clinicians can make decisions about oxygen requirements (Everitt et al., 2021).

Sleep apnoea is another reason that some children may require respiratory support at home. This is a potentially serious sleep disorder that causes pauses in breathing during sleep. There are many risk factors for it, including certain underlying conditions. If a child is suspected of having central, obstructive, or complex sleep apnoea, this will be diagnosed with a sleep study and a continuous positive airway pressure (CPAP) mask will be supplied for use overnight (NICE, 2021). The disadvantage of CPAP is that it is loud and many people find it uncomfortable (it's like breathing in when a gale force wind is blowing in your face). For this reason, some trials are testing positional devices (Xiao et al., 2021) and humidified high-flow nasal cannula oxygen (Wong et al., 2021), which appears to be better tolerated, but these are not standard treatments in the UK.

The number of children requiring long-term ventilation (LTV) in the UK has increased significantly, and many of these children are cared for at home (Wallis et al., 2011). Children may be ventilated via a non-invasive mask, or by tracheostomy, and this might be continuously, or just overnight depending on the child's condition. They may require tracheostomy tube changes at home, suctioning, or monitoring. Respiratory support often feels overwhelming to families initially, and the key to them feeling more confident is having the information and education they need about equipment, emergency protocols, and daily care.

Why Childhood Illness Matters

Feeding support

Feeding is an important part of healthcare and recovery, and ensuring that children get optimal nutrition and hydration while they are unwell can be a challenge. There are many ways that children may be fed while they are unwell, depending on their age, and their condition.

Oral feeding: whenever possible, it is encouraged to feed children orally to promote normality, reduce the risk of feeding dysfunction, and because this is more acceptable to families as well as being more cost-effective and efficient. This means that if a child has a safe and effective swallow, and is able to consume sufficient nutrients to sustain their growth and development orally, then this should continue. Children may be exclusively orally fed, or they may be partially orally fed and supplemented with enteral feeds – this will depend on many factors including their growth, nutrition needs and condition. The type of oral feeding will obviously depend on the child's age. Children who need support with oral feeding either because of dysphagia or insufficient calorie intake will be seen and assessed by a speech and language therapist and dietitian for specific individual advice and support, but an infant feeding specialist (ideally with clinical paediatric experience) can also be a great source of information and support alongside a child's clinical care.

Breastfeeding: it is recommended to breastfeed exclusively for the first six months, and to continue alongside solid foods until the child is at least two years old. There is no age at which breastmilk ceases to be individually tailored nutritionally, and it continues to provide immunological benefit for as long as the mother and child breastfeed. However, all that said, breastfeeding sick children can present many challenges and specific support for sick children in paediatrics is not always easy to find because current training mostly covers the healthy population and preterm infants, rather than sick children beyond the neonatal period. There is more information about breastfeeding sick children in *Breastfeeding the Brave* (Hookway, 2022).

Formula feeding: formula feeding can also be challenging for sick children who may have poor appetite, nausea, or may be excessively sleepy and fatigued. Support may be given by a speech and language therapist, as well as a dietitian. Formula feeds may also be given in addition to breastfeeds for some children – for example if they have very high calorie needs but need a small volume of fluid, which can be a difficult combination. General information about formula feeding, including safety and practical points, is covered in *Why Formula Feeding Matters* (Banks, 2022).

Solids: solid food intake, unsurprisingly, is also affected by illness and certain conditions. However, eating solids provides an opportunity for developmentally normal mouth and jaw movements, social interaction, pleasure, and sensory experiences. Whenever possible and safe, children with medical complexity are encouraged to eat the family's usual diet. Some modifications to solids may be required, such as mashing or chopping into small pieces. Solids gradually replace exclusive milk feeds in a developmentally and nutritionally appropriate way, with the introduction of solids at six months continuing to be the global recommendation. More information about the importance of starting solids can be found in *Why Starting Solids Matters* (Brown, 2017).

Enteral feeding: when children cannot meet their nutritional requirements to maintain growth, or cannot do this safely, they may be partially or exclusively enterally fed. This means liquid nutrition is given via a tube into the stomach. Digestion still occurs in the stomach and intestinal tract but bypasses the mouth – which is essential in children with an unsafe swallow, or reduced consciousness, as well as those who cannot tolerate oral feeds, have severe nausea, or cannot maintain their growth. Enteral feeding is usually preferable, if possible, to parenteral feeding as it preserves gastrointestinal function, is safer, and simpler (Braegger et al., 2010). Enteral feeds are usually liquid ready-to-use preparations based on cow's milk with added fibre, vitamins, and minerals, but sometimes a specialised product is needed – for example for children with allergy, short gut, chylothorax, liver disease, high calorie needs or malabsorption. The feeds are given either as a bolus (measured doses every few hours) or continuously, and there are clinically compelling reasons why one approach may be chosen over another.

Nasogastric tube: this is a thin silicone tube that is passed through one of the child's nostrils, or less frequently their mouth, via the oesophagus into the top of the child's stomach. It is measured and passed by a nurse, or a parent who has been trained to position the tube. It does not hurt to pass a nasogastric (NG) or orogastric (OG) tube, but it is uncomfortable and moreover, the tube needs to be changed fairly frequently, and stuck down on the cheek. Some tubes can remain in situ for up to eight weeks, but many need changing every 3–5 days. The repeated sticking of the tube can be painful on the child's skin (Fumarola et al., 2020), so the nostril side is alternated. However, although many infants and children get used to their tube, others are prone to pulling it out, or gagging when it is passed. They are therefore not suitable for long-term use. Some children have a nasojejunal tube, which is passed further into the intestine and bypasses the stomach completely – these are not suitable for a parent to pass as their position needs to be confirmed by X-ray.

PEG tube: if enteral feeding is expected to be long term, a gastrostomy is usually recommended. This is a surgically inserted button in the stomach to allow feeds to be connected via a tube and is indicated for significant feeding challenges that are long term. The incidence of percutaneous endoscopic gastrostomy (PEG) tubes is rising and the average age of insertion is falling among children (Homan et al., 2021). The decision to site a PEG is obviously one that requires a multidisciplinary and family-centred approach. The PEG requires observation by the parent for signs of infection, and needs daily care as well as training to use it for feeds. Although a PEG can be a life-saving intervention, there are associated negative impacts on quality of life (Glasson et al., 2020) and parents may need emergency information about what to do if their child's gastrostomy button becomes dislodged.

Total Parenteral Nutrition (TPN): some children require TPN at home. This is intravenous nutrition administered through a central line (a long-term IV line such as a Hickman or Port-a-cath) and may be indicated for children with benign or malignant disease with chronic intestinal failure, or significant malnutrition – in other words, for children who are unable to meet their nutritional requirements with oral or enteral nutrition. Clearly the decision to provide TPN long-term is not one that is taken lightly, and the risks of TPN need to be weighed against the benefits – for example, the child has to be metabolically stable, as TPN bypasses intestinal absorption and is metabolised by the liver, the home environment needs to be safe, and the parent needs to be fully informed and educated on how to administer the TPN, including the use of the central line. TPN administration also requires collaboration between the parent, doctor, nurse, dietitian, and pharmacist (Pironi et al., 2020). As you might imagine, interventions like TPN can be frightening, overwhelming, and exhausting for parents (Page et al., 2020).

Skin care

Children with long-term conditions, receiving certain interventions, or those with reduced mobility, are more at risk of skin breakdown. Those with wounds, devices, catheters, central lines, tracheostomies, stomas and so on have a higher risk of infection and those who have limited independent movement are at risk of pressure sores caused by pressure and friction (Triantafyllou et al., 2021). Parents may have some support from community nursing teams and tissue viability nurses who will visit at home, but they are likely to need to care for their child's skin on a daily basis. The type of skin and wound care will also be affected by the age of the child, as neonatal skin care presents unique challenges (Steen et al., 2020).

Parents or carers may also need to care for their child's bladder and bowel function. Almost all parents use nappies when their children are infants and very young toddlers, but some children with additional needs or medical complexity may have continence needs for many years, which means their skin will be exposed to urine and faeces with an additional threat to skin integrity. Other children may have stoma bags that collect urine or faeces (and sometimes both). Some parents report anxiety around caring for and cleaning these devices – fearing that they may tear the skin and tissues (Page et al., 2020).

Specialist nurses and occupational therapists may be able to advise on and provide specialist equipment such as pressure-relieving mattresses, chairs, mobility equipment, home adaptations and postural and positioning devices and support. If a family is struggling, it is always a good idea to ask for a review of their care to see if there is any additional product, device, service, or therapy that might help.

Joined-up care

Collaboration of professionals is obviously necessary to achieve the best outcomes for these remarkable families (Luzi et al., 2019). Collaboration avoids the situation where a family needs to retell their story several times, fall through cracks in services, or be forced to fill in those gaps left by patchy service provision. The best models are those where hospital and community services have good liaison between:

- Lead paediatrician
- Respiratory specialists
- Community children's nursing team
- Pain team
- Hospice
- Palliative care teams
- Social worker
- Health visitor or school nurse

Families frequently express a wish to be given enough information by the right person to make a decision, and this includes peer-to-peer support so that parents can hear from other parents with lived experience (Peat et al., 2023).

A recent review (Brenner et al., 2019) found numerous practical things that make a difference including:

- A designated lead clinician who can take responsibility and get to know a family well
- Continuity of care facilitated by digital records
- Technical support at home for equipment and machinery
- Parents have adequate training to ensure they feel confident with their child's clinical care needs
- Sibling and parent psychological support as standard
- Access to community pharmacists
- Children having access to preventative and public health services including developmental checks and dental care
- Transportation that is suitable for technology-dependent children
- Information provided at a level that is cognitively and culturally appropriate for families
- Direct access to a paediatric emergency department and PICU
- Access to hospice and respite services when required
- Joined-up handover of care from paediatric services to adult services
- Discharge and transfer planning to ensure care is continuous and safe
- Appropriate intervention from allied therapies

Although this is obviously mindbogglingly complex to organise, evidence suggests that achieving this type of care is associated with fewer emergency and intensive care admissions (Perez-Jolles et al., 2019). Effective collaborative care ensures high-quality and compassionate service provision for children, but it does practically speaking mean that parents or carers have to become experts at handling logistics and coordinating all the appointments their child needs. They also need to find time to complete any exercises, give the medications that their child needs, take their children to rehabilitative sessions and see various therapists. All of this is of course in addition to providing all the non-clinical care, social and educational opportunities and play that their child needs, as well as care for any other children, and looking after themselves.

Emotional, psychological, and practical support

By now it should be obvious that the mental load of parents of children with medical complexity is often high. It is little wonder that many studies find that although joy and a sense of privilege is prevalent, so too is stress. If you are just getting to know a family, ask them what they need, rather than make assumptions. Many parents can give you a full breakdown of their child's condition, strengths, preferences, needs, challenges, and any treatments. What they are often sorely in need of is a break! It can feel scary and stressful to entrust a child with medical needs to someone else, so allow plenty of time for them to be able to brief you on the essential details and make sure you feel clear on your role and responsibilities as well. Remember that parents of children with complex needs are highly skilled and experienced, and will be able to tell you everything you need to know about their child. The hard part for them may be the ability to switch off.

Positive language

While I have acknowledged that caring for sick children can be hard work, many parents work hard to ensure that their child is spoken about with compassion and dignity. Failing to use skilled, compassionate language can cause parents profound distress and make a difficult situation harder to handle.

> *'I have confronted my own ableism around how I dealt with my son's diagnosis. Often, a media narrative*

portrays Disabled people as burdens and their caregivers as heroic figures sacrificing themselves. I know this fed into my fears but looking back, a huge part of how I responded was also shaped by how that diagnosis was delivered. In a few minutes, two people who had never met anyone with bilateral perisylvian polymicrogyria told us what not to expect from our son, with no ongoing psychological support. No wonder I was scared. No wonder I felt hopeless. No wonder it took me years to heal those wounds.

I've thought a lot about what would have helped me when receiving my son's diagnosis. It would have been helpful if the doctors acknowledged the psychological impact that this news would likely have on us. We were entering a process of grief, but what made it worse was that we didn't recognise it. This took a lot of energy to work through, a lot of questioning and guilt, and this all took energy away from supporting our son.

Offering signposting of support would have helped us; from immediate support for families within the hospital to information about ongoing psychological support (EMDR therapy helped me immensely once I discovered it), to support for us as a couple since our marriage was likely to (and did) take a hit. Accessing this support early would have saved me from expending energy climbing out of the darkness and experiencing poor mental health. Being emotionally well has allowed me to be a better caregiver to my son. So that should be a priority.

Signposting to other families who had a similar experience would have helped immensely. There are many organisations that offer this, but we didn't know about any of them and were so overwhelmed that we didn't think to look. What we needed was understanding,

> *a shared lived experience, and hope. If I could teleport back to that room, on the day of my son's diagnosis, I would tell myself, "It's going to be hard, but a strength has been born in you today that will never stop growing. You can do hard things." I would also say "your son's diagnosis feels like it will be life-defining to him and you, but it won't be. What will define your lives is the love you have for each other and the strength you share".*
>
> *Secondly, what would have helped would be to hear a balanced diagnosis. I wouldn't define my son by the list of things he can't do; I would define him by the light he brings into any room, by his infectious laugh, by his tenacity. I believe all professionals should be educated in, and use, the social model of disability, which highlights that disability primarily results from societal barriers, rather than inherent flaws in the individual. This shift could empower healthcare professionals to deliver medical information, empathy, and optimism, honouring each individual's potential.'* Shurron Rosales

If you work with people with disability, you can read more about the social model of disability (Oliver, 1983), which fundamentally asserts that people are not disabled by their impairments but by the disabling conditions within society.

Advocating for children

At times, parents may need to be their child's champion and voice. Happily, most healthcare professionals are sincere, highly trained, eminently capable, and extremely compassionate. Even so, sometimes parents may feel like their gut instinct is telling them something is wrong, or that an aspect of their child's care has been overlooked. It's always okay to speak up if you feel concerns are not being addressed, or you're worried something has been missed.

All of us are human, and not only that, but parents are the world experts on their children. Paediatric healthcare professionals are undoubtedly the best people to deal with illness and medical complexity, but nobody knows a child like their parents do. This means that while the clinicians may understand the illness or condition better, they may not understand how the illness manifests in *this* child. Of course there is a fine line here between trusting healthcare professionals blindly, and appropriately challenging in the process of advocacy. Sometimes the clinicians really *are* right. Other times they're not. Figuring out which way round it is isn't always easy and can lead to anxiety and sometimes chasing a diagnosis that doesn't exist.

I remember being transferred to a specialist cancer hospital for a bone marrow biopsy for our daughter. Upon arrival she rapidly perked up and started jumping on the bed. The doctors smiled in a relieved way, thinking that she couldn't possibly have leukaemia because the bone pain that is usual on presentation would inhibit such joyful casual trampolining. Of course, she *did* have leukaemia, and I had to advocate for my daughter on several occasions when she *appeared* well, but I knew she wasn't.

The bottom line is that if a parent remains concerned, they should seek further input until they feel resolution has been found.

Palliative care

Sadly, some children have conditions which are either life-limiting or become terminal, and this book would unfortunately be incomplete without an acknowledgement of this devastating fact. Palliative care should be integrated into paediatric care when a child receives a life-limiting diagnosis

(Weaver et al., 2015) and should continue irrespective of whether a child receives treatment that is targeted at the disease – in other words, palliative care is not just about managing pain and making a child comfortable (Nilsson et al., 2020). Palliative care is also related to symptom management, providing compassionate counselling to family members, and discussing options for end-of-life care including tough decisions about where a child may die.

None of this is easy to read (or frankly to write) but as I was once taught as a junior nurse – death is a meaningful part of life. Caring for children at the end of their life is something that anyone working with children with complex needs must be prepared for. However, to give you a lived experience version of this highly emotive topic, I am indebted to Hannah Chapman, the bereaved mother of Maisie, who died just before she was six months old, from mitochondrial disease.

> What was really helpful to Hannah and her family
>
> We were told by a very brave doctor that she didn't think Maisie was going to live very long. It must have been an impossible task when Maisie was currently undiagnosed, and medical staff like to be certain of things before giving bad news, but we are utterly thankful that she did. It gave us the ability to prepare and begin our grieving process.
>
> Immediately after diagnosis we didn't have time to break down and cry. The reality was we had Maisie's two-year old brother, Lowen, to look after as well, and he pulled me to do a dinosaur puzzle in the playroom, while my husband Ben remained in Maisie's hospital room. Lowen has unknowingly pulled us out of our grief ever

since. We were – and continue to be – so very lucky to have him.

How we coped when we knew her condition was terminal
We coped in those early days of diagnosis as best we could. Gulps of red wine before bed, breaking the news to friends and family and spending as much time as possible together as a family. I would just stare at Maisie, terrified of the pain of the future, trying to memorise every inch of her for my future self. I took lots of photos and videos, danced and sang with her, and just held her, stroking her hands. I also desperately needed to find others who had been there and survived it. When you google 'bereaved parents' all you tend to find is unhelpful quotes about the unbearable pain. Not having a diagnosis made this hard. There were no charities or online forums to turn to. And because of a miscommunication between the hospitals, our local hospital didn't provide us with any emotional support either. I turned to Instagram and the growing baby loss community and eventually found my lifesavers, the most wonderful, brave parents who had or were going through it.

We decided to do all we could with the short life that Maisie had. We wrote a bucket list for her of things we'd like to show her and places to take her – and this gave us something positive to focus on. We introduced her to family and friends, had a Thanksgiving service, went to festivals, holidays, picnics – along with giving her endless bubble baths, kisses, and cuddles.

What I'd have wanted ideally
I would have much preferred her to have died in a hospice. Her death in hospital, surrounded by strangers,

bright lights, and a scary environment was the opposite of what I would have hoped for. Although death isn't necessarily easy, it may have been a little more controlled. And we would have been able to stay with her as much as we would have liked. I wish that children never had to go to a mortuary. Ideally they should be cared for within a hospice, or family room in a hospital, where they can be cared for as much or as little as the family would like. I hated having to make appointments to see my daughter, and I wish I could have cared for her more myself. I wanted to be the one to bathe and clothe her rather than a stranger.

But we were also able to do some memory-making in the hospital after she died. Doing hand and footprints, changing her clothes one last time, singing to her and giving her cuddles.

How I handled my grief immediately
The first days after Maisie died were a blur. Those days involved support from our local hospice. I cuddled Lowen as much as he would let me (the oxytocin coursing through my veins felt like it was healing me). I went to visit Maisie every day I was allowed to. We lit candles – they burned all night long. We bought picture frames and put photos of Maisie in every room of the house (even the bathroom and car). We continued to make her monthly birthday cakes and sing to her.

What helped us
Grief is an incredibly personal thing. It's as individual as the relationship you have with the person that is gone. But I coped with a few activities:

- Fundraising for charities – it gave Maisie's death some

meaning
- Running – we have run many races in Maisie's name
- Writing
- Sharing my grief journey online, and sharing her pictures
- Putting a bench on a very special hill overlooking the sea (made by Maisie's Granddad)
- Making a book called *Yellow Day* about my grief
- Taking up gardening and growing many, many flowers

When we were originally given Maisie's diagnosis, we felt incredibly powerless. The only thing we could really control was how we dealt with it. So I decided to view everything as positively as possible – to try to be thankful for the days we did have. It wasn't easy, but it was my way of coping, and this continued after her death.

How grief changed over time
I've always found that grief comes in waves – initially they are huge stormy waves – but you learn to ride the big waves, remembering they will subside eventually. Now the waves aren't as noticeable, but they are always there in the background, and one can still come out of nowhere, knocking you right back to those first waves of grief.

Tips for parents facing a terminal diagnosis
- Try not to have regrets. Do all the things you want to do now. Lots of fun, happy memory-making
- Take as many photos, and especially videos, as you can
- Contact people who have been through it – get help, find your people to get you through
- Have faith that you can survive this. It seems

- impossible – but your love for your child will get you through
- Find positive ways to keep your child's memory alive
- Hold on to your memories – as not even death can take them from you

When I went to visit Maisie for the last time, the day before her funeral, I drove to the funeral directors' alone. I spent over an hour with her, kissing her head, stroking her hair, talking, and singing, I never wanted to leave. I made a promise to her. I told her that when I was strong enough, I was going to live again – for her. I was going to smile and laugh, I was going to do good things and help others. I was going to do all those incredible world-changing things that she was meant to do. I believe that is my purpose – I need to lead two lives now – to make her impact felt on the world. I have lots of ideas – and I am making them happen, bit by tiny bit.

7

Childhood illness and sleep

By now, you've probably accepted that even if children do not have a serious or chronic illness, getting sick is basically a fact of life. Coughs, colds, stomach bugs, earaches, and fevers – you can virtually guarantee that by the age of two years, most children will have had their fair share of illness. They have immature immune systems (Simon et al., 2015) and develop their immunity through exposure to a wide variety of germs (Greaves, 2006; Urayama et al., 2010; Zachek et al., 2015). They also mix with other little people who have similarly immature immune systems and poor awareness of hygiene and infection control, so they generously share whatever they have with anyone in a two-metre radius.

That's before we consider the children who are born prematurely, those with congenital anomalies that make them medically complex, children with other vulnerabilities or children who develop critical or chronic illness which leads to many months or years of treatment, hospitalisation, and medical care.

Childhood illness and sleep

It's fair to say, then, that most children will have some experience of illness, to a greater or lesser extent, and this is likely to lead to sleep disruption. This in turn is likely to lead to parents asking for help with their child's sleep. Many people ask me for advice about sleep when a child is sick or has been diagnosed with a condition or disability. The questions normally fall into three categories:

1. Does condition X cause sleep problems and if so, *what* sleep problems?
2. What sleep strategies will work given they are unwell?
3. How can we minimise sleep disruption during illness?

Of course, it is impossible to cover the ways in which every condition affects sleep in this book. The truth is that often illness affects sleep in a fairly generic way (pain and discomfort affects how we sleep) but there are specific nuances as well. If a child has an underlying condition, it is *always* appropriate to ensure that they are receiving all the usual medical care they need. There may be some supportive strategies that parents can consider in parallel to managing illness, but it really depends on how acutely unwell they are. This chapter will outline the ways in which sleep is affected by illness, the different effects on sleep with mild, self-limiting illness, serious or chronic illness and disability, and how to navigate sleep through illness. I will also cover the impact of responsive parenting and family-centred care on parental confidence and self-esteem, because failing to honour this has been found to be a significant stressor associated with sleep practices in hospital.

How does illness impact sleep?

Let's start with mild and self-limiting illnesses. These include the usual repertoire of coughs, colds, diarrhoea and vomiting bugs, earaches, and fevers. The most common illnesses are the upper respiratory tract infections (URTIs) which cause symptoms of cough, sore throat, runny nose, headache, fever, and reduced appetite. While these symptoms are usually mild, they can have a profound effect on a child's behaviour and sleep. Many children will get over an URTI within two weeks, though the acute phase with maximum sleep disruption is usually shorter than that. URTIs disrupt sleep because a child usually feels generally unwell, coughs, and may have a fever. They may also mouth-breathe, which causes a dry mouth and usually results in waking more for a drink, as well as comfort.

Gastroenteritis can strike with little warning, spreads rapidly around childcare settings and usually causes intense, though mercifully brief, disruption. Not only are children usually awake at night with stomach cramps, nausea, vomiting and diarrhoea, but they may also have disruption to feeding, drinking and eating, and they might have a fever. It's obvious that for most little ones with gastroenteritis, sleep will be minimal.

Earaches are extremely painful, and unfortunately, young children are particularly prone to them because their eustachian tube is immature and the more horizontal position of it makes fluid build-up more likely. Lying down, especially on the affected side, can be very painful, and that's without any other symptoms, such as fever or an associated URTI.

I won't name every illness individually that can affect sleep because it's hopefully obvious that anything that is uncomfortable, painful, inconvenient, or distressing in the day will also cause problems at night. A good tip is to get organised for the night ahead: make sure that drinks, a thermometer, medications, tissues, cloths, sick buckets, spare bedding, and anything else that might be required, are nearby.

Childhood illness and sleep

Managing sleep during acute illness

I wish there was a way to avoid sleep problems during illness, but I would be lying if I said there was. It's been my experience over the years that when a child is more seriously unwell, or if a child has a fever, they tend to respond by sleeping more, either by napping more than usual, going to bed earlier, or sleeping more solidly at night. However, many children with mild illnesses, or in the recovery phase of illness, will have much more disrupted sleep. For the most part, parents will need to accept that for the duration of the illness, a child will have increased night-time needs, and sleep disruption is inevitable. It is usually possible to tell when the acute phase of an illness has passed, and the recovery phase has started. Once the main symptom (whether that's fever, vomiting or obvious pain) has stopped or substantially improved, it's usually safe to assume that while the child is still probably not feeling great, they are beginning to get better.

Once recovering, parents usually want to begin to get back on track, but this needs to be realistic. A child will often require a lot of input while they are bored, cranky, uncomfortable, or experiencing reduced appetite. While they may need less intense input when they are recovering, they will not be ready to get back to their usual sleeping pattern either. They may have napped more in the day, which can sometimes result in less sleep at night – after all, there's only so much sleep you can achieve in 24 hours!

Some practical tips include trying to keep some elements of a familiar bedtime routine going if this is appropriate, as well as staying on top of symptoms such as pain and fever to reduce discomfort-related waking.

Sleep and chronic illness

While it is obvious that sleep may be a distant memory during acute illness, this is harder to deal with when an illness or condition lasts for more than just a few days. Children with chronic health problems often have trouble with sleep. This may be due to needing medication or monitoring at night, increased symptoms at night, disruption to routines due to medications or hospitalisation, or anxiety (Hysing et al., 2009). These sleep problems include more difficulty falling asleep, staying asleep, and waking earlier in the morning. Children with cerebral palsy are more likely to have sleep problems compared to typically developing peers, and sleep problems are worse in children who are less mobile (Hulst et al., 2021; 2022). Children with asthma are more likely to have disturbed sleep due to worsened symptoms at night (Kavanagh et al., 2018) and the possible association between asthma and sleep-disordered breathing (Castro-Rodriguez et al., 2017). Eczema is known to cause significant problems with sleep and daytime functioning (Camfferman et al., 2010). Diabetes has been shown to be linked with challenges at bedtime and insomnia (Monaghan et al., 2012) and these sleep problems are known to cause stress (Bassi et al., 2021). Neurological disorders such as epilepsy and traumatic brain injury are similarly found to cause sleep disturbance (Dorris et al., 2008), and cancers are known to cause many sleep problems for several reasons (Walter et al., 2015), with these effects persisting after treatment has ended (van Deuren et al., 2020). Meanwhile, children with critical illness in intensive care are often given medications that cause sedation but paradoxically reduce the quality of sleep, particularly deep sleep (Kudchadkar et al., 2014).

This is before we consider sleep pathology such as sleep-disordered breathing, and obstructive and central sleep apnoea (see Chapter 6). There has recently been an explosion of interest in mouth-breathing, which has a complex aetiology and may be caused by genetics, allergy, recurrent respiratory infections, deviated septum, adenoid/tonsil hypertrophy, low tone, poor sleep position, malocclusion or not breastfeeding (Tomaz et al., 2012; Jimenez et al., 2015; Zhao et al., 2021). Exactly how to treat children with mouth-breathing in the absence of underlying pathology remains unclear, but certainly it would be sensible to ensure children are seen by a paediatrician, ENT surgeon, dentist or speech and language therapist as appropriate.

One recent study suggested that 'lax' parenting behaviours (defined as bedsharing, providing food and drink in the bedroom, offering comfort in the night) could be an explanation for the poorer sleep seen in children with acute lymphoblastic leukaemia compared to healthy controls (McCarthy et al., 2016). Of course, this ignores the fact that children with cancer experience anxiety, discomfort, pain, and medication side effects – all of which would arguably be more solid explanations for worsening sleep than so-called 'lax' parenting. Another study promoted the use of non-responsive sleep training involving leaving children to cry without parental reassurance or support while in hospital and about to undergo stem cell transplant (LaRosa et al., 2021). Regardless of your position on cry-it-out sleep training, most people would agree that a non-responsive approach to sleep management at a time when a sick child is likely to be scared and uncomfortable is pretty hard-core. Not only is this likely to cause stress for a child and their family, but it is loud and disruptive to other families on the hospital ward as well! Personally, I would never recommend an approach to sleep that ignores a child's need for prompt, attuned caregiving.

Just as with acute illness, any uncomfortable symptom can disrupt sleep, but clearly for children with more chronic health conditions this can be more problematic, so it is harder to justify an 'anything goes' policy when this could result in chronic and severe sleep deprivation for both parents and children. Therefore, it is even more important for these children that they have the right treatment, management and supports in place to reduce sleep-disrupting symptoms – whether that is pain relief, supportive wedges, and cushions to reduce muscle cramps, correcting anaemia, referring for sleep pathology, medications to support sleep, or timing procedures or drugs that disrupt sleep better, to name but a few (Hookway, 2021).

Sleep and stress

Sleep is a feature of the parasympathetic nervous system. This is often called the 'rest and digest' state. When we are alert, stressed, anxious, nervous, uncomfortable, frightened or in pain, our sympathetic nervous system is activated – often known as the 'fight or flight' response. This is over-simplifying though, because the sympathetic nervous system is not just activated during times when we need to run away, but also at any time when we are alert, active and concentrating. The relevance for illness is probably obvious – if a child or their family is frightened or stressed, or the child is in pain or uncomfortable, the sympathetic nervous system is activated, and sleep will be more difficult or impossible.

The solution is to be aware of times when the child is obviously alert and focused, and not to try to coax sleep at times when this is physiologically not likely to happen. Similarly, at times when they are sore, stressed, sick or scared, sleep is unlikely, so focus on addressing the problem at hand, rather than trying to explain to a child how important rest and sleep are for healing – this is not helpful!

Childhood illness and sleep

Hospitalisation and sleep

For children who are more seriously unwell, admission to hospital is sometimes necessary. Hospitalisation, while enabling appropriate monitoring, clinical intervention and management of various illnesses and conditions, brings with it a whole new level of disruption to sleep, as well as to parenting and the family unit. My research in 2022 found that various aspects of responsive parenting, bedsharing and sleep were exceptionally challenging for many families (Hookway et al., 2023).

The main issues within the context of sleep and family life reported by families include:

- Lack of flexibility with bedsharing
- Poor awareness of the interplay between breastfeeding and bedsharing
- Mothers feeling they had to choose between breastfeeding and sleep
- Difficulty sleeping in parent pull-out beds
- Inaccurate advice about night feeding and sleep
- Trauma
- Disruption to family life, including separation from siblings and partners

Bedsharing, breastfeeding and sleep

Bedsharing is culturally normal in many parts of the world (McKenna et al., 2007). Sharing sleep locations is practised from birth by the global majority, and many parents choose this option from birth. Bedsharing is practised because it usually facilitates easier settling of young infants and children, provides reassurance and comfort, facilitates easier breastfeeding and faster return to sleep, and because many people find it enjoyable (McKenna and Gettler, 2016).

Bedsharing is also known to be associated with longer durations of breastfeeding (Ball et al., 2016).

Bedsharing is the subject of considerable controversy, largely due to western-centric ideals of promoting early solo sleeping, and because of confusing messaging about Sudden Infant Death Syndrome (SIDS). It is frequently painted as not only a 'bad habit', but a risky one at that, despite data showing that it is *unsafe* bedsharing (including sofa sleeping) which increases the rate of SIDS, rather than bedsharing in a manner that is not known to increase risk (Zimmerman et al., 2023; Blair et al., 2020).

Bedsharing in hospital

Bedsharing in hospital is obviously a more difficult scenario to consider, due to patients with unknown, as well as known, vulnerabilities, the difficulty of a child being in bed with an adult when healthcare professionals may need to attend to the child easily overnight, and other issues. Hospital floors are hard, beds are sometimes high off the ground, and there are tubes, lines, and wires to become entangled in. Some children also have evolving conditions, reduced neurological status, or are at risk of rapid deterioration. For these reasons and more I have a huge amount of sympathy for the headache that this creates in terms of creating nuanced guidelines that both keep sick children safer, and aim to facilitate breastfeeding, responsive parenting and making comforting those children easier.

Bedsharing using side-car cribs has been studied on the postnatal ward, and no adverse incidents were observed (Ball et al., 2006); however, the paediatric population is very different from the maternity population, where infants are newborn and largely healthy. Quite apart from the fact that sick children in paediatrics may have evolving and unstable

Childhood illness and sleep

conditions, they are often larger and physically do not fit in a side-car crib.

What I know from my own clinical experience, as the mother of a sick child, and from my research in this area, is that children who usually bedshare do not find solo sleep easy. They especially do not find it easy when they are sick, scared and in an unfamiliar place with sensory overload. This means that if those children are placed in cots or cribs alone, unless they are seriously unwell and have reduced responsiveness, they protest. Loudly. This means less sleep for them, their resident parent, and frankly the whole ward.

From a practical point of view, it also means that many parents bring their child into the pull-out parent bed or convertible chair bed. These are usually much narrower, flimsier, and harder for staff to access. In short – the risks they are trying to avoid are instead magnified. One pragmatic option is to provide a single patient bed with a bedrail instead, but this does of course depend on the child's condition.

Managing a child who usually bedshares, but cannot

It is important to remember that for a family who bedshares, there will be important and meaningful reasons why they choose this approach to sleep. Being unable to bedshare for a genuine clinical reason may therefore be a loss, present inconvenience, or cause distress.

Firstly, approach this with an open mind. Is bedsharing truly not an option? What is the clinical rationale for avoiding bedsharing in this situation? It may be obvious, but other clinical scenarios are less cut and dried, and some open-mindedness may be needed.

Secondly, demonstrate compassion to families. This includes withholding judgement on their bedsharing preference, but also showing that you understand this is difficult for them. It often really helps parents to know what the clinical justification for avoiding bedsharing is. For example, is this child likely to rapidly deteriorate and the healthcare team are concerned that if they need to urgently intervene it would present a risk to their care? Having a reason is often helpful when something meaningful is taken away.

Thirdly, try to find ways to make this easier. Are there compromises? For example, could the child be fed or cuddled to sleep on a large bed, and then placed in the cot/crib once they are asleep? Could a single hospital bed be provided in addition to a cot, rather than a cot and a parent pull-out bed?

Finally, if the child's condition changes, or stabilises, could bedsharing be an option again? In essence, can we keep the decision-making about bedsharing fluid, rather than fixed?

Supporting sleep in hospital

If a child does not bedshare, or it is felt to be too risky to bedshare, then there are many ways to facilitate more rest for children, including:

- Maintaining their usual bedtime routines if possible
- Dimming the lights
- Bringing familiar comfort objects to hospital
- Reading bedtime stories
- Ensuring they have adequate pain relief before bed
- Arranging their medication to facilitate more consolidated stretches of sleep
- Avoiding prescribing at night unless it is clinically essential

The medication part of the puzzle is particularly important. This does not just mean topping up analgesia, but also avoiding prescribing medication that might be stimulating prior to sleep. Using some common sense overnight to avoid excessively interrupting sleep and rest is hugely appreciated by families. For example, if the clinical observations are due at 10pm, 2am and 6am, and IV drugs have to be given at midnight and 4am, this means that the family will be interrupted every two hours all night. While nursing routines can become habitual and task-orientated, there is no clinical reason why the observations cannot happen at the same time as the IV medications to avoid disturbing the child and family twice the number of times. Equally, is there a rationale for checking the child's clinical observations every four hours? Or could they be left for six hours? There cannot be a blanket answer to this question because children's needs should be clinically assessed – but it's always worth asking the question and hoping for some open-minded and flexible practice.

Family-centred approaches to sleep

I'm a passionate advocate of family-centred care because we can care best for children when we care about their families as well. Given that parents are partners in care, we cannot expect them to care as effectively, or without considerable cost to themselves, if they are not rested. Optimising the whole family's sleep, whether on the paediatric ward or at home, is *part* of family-centred care (Hookway, 2021).

So, what does family-centred sleep during illness look like?

Considering the whole family: no child exists in a bubble. Is there a healthy sibling who needs to be considered? Does this child only settle for one parent? What is the impact of the child's illness on the parent who is resident with them? Is there anything practical that could be considered to support the family? Is having two beds an option to allow siblings to stay?

Honouring their sleep traditions: of course, medical emergencies can and do happen, and the child's health and wellbeing is always paramount. However, many hospital stays include disruptions that are avoidable. Could the family have a 'do not disturb' time so bedtime can proceed uninterrupted by ward rounds, medications, or clinical observations? Could they be afforded some privacy so that they can get undressed and ready for bed without fear of someone walking in suddenly? Preserving some of these aspects of normality can go a long way towards supporting a family's functioning.

Negotiate shared care: many parents of children with long-term health needs are used to caring for their child's medical needs at night. Some children require medication, monitoring or feeding at night. For some parents, it is disempowering to have these roles removed from them. Just because they are in hospital, these tasks do not necessarily have to be undertaken by clinical staff if the family usually attends to them. On the other hand, they may really appreciate a break and a chance to sleep. The only way to know is to negotiate this open-mindedly.

Individualised risk assessment: rather than have a one-size-fits-all approach to many aspects of overnight care, such as frequency of observation/monitoring, medications, and bedsharing, it is arguably more sensitive as well as more appropriate to individually risk-assess each situation. Perhaps bedsharing or adjusting medication timings isn't appropriate for every family, but it may be suitable for some.

Self-aware care: this is an aspect of nursing care that is not taught, but it is intuitive to many. It is the practice of consciously wondering how a clinician's practice might affect

Childhood illness and sleep

a family, and how, with modifications to a clinician's style of working, they can make a family's life easier. For example, offering to change nappies overnight, being considerate when using lights and torches overnight, and wearing quiet shoes. It also includes going the extra mile – nurses can set alarms so they know when an IV infusion will end, so they can be there ready for it, preventing the pump from alarming.

Being noise aware: on a closely related point, hospitals are noisy places. There are many things that can be done to minimise noise – such as silencing observation machines before entering rooms and open bays, promptly attending to alarming devices and monitoring equipment, not taking phone calls or talking to colleagues in the open bay, and silencing bleeps promptly.

Trauma and stress-informed practice: part of family-centred care is accepting that parents and families are likely to be stressed, anxious or traumatised. They may not only have their own concerns about their child and the diagnosis, but adults are also likely to have other stressors, such as work, finances, partners, and any existing mental health challenges of their own. Being in hospital with a sick child makes accessing usual sources of support challenging or impossible, and it can be lonely and isolating. All of this can raise stress levels and inhibit sleep.

Sleep recovery after hospital admission

Once a child is discharged from hospital, from either an acute one-off admission, or simply until their next recurrent admission to hospital, there will inevitably be a few days of getting back into a normal rhythm. This may mean that the first day or two will feel more chaotic than usual, or that there are problems with settling or getting back to usual routines, naps, or bedtimes.

Children may also have anxiety or experience ongoing pain or discomfort which may raise their stress levels – again, this will inhibit sleep. Focusing on the underlying causes, managing anxiety, and providing comfort and reassurance, are all immediately obvious ways to manage the transition back to home.

From a practical point of view, staying calm, lowering expectations, and making life as easy as possible for parents are all pragmatic ways to cope. Tensions can often run high, especially when there is a degree of sleep deprivation, so taking shifts if there are two parents around, and getting some early nights, can also help to bank some sleep.

Finally, for families of children who have ongoing healthcare needs, sleep should be part of the care plan and therefore assessed at regular intervals. However, these conversations need to be nuanced and individualised, making sure that questions around sleep are asked in a respectful way. Families who are asked about their child's sleep, the impact their care needs have on their adult sleep, and whether they have any concerns about sleep, are more likely to describe a positive interaction than families who are *told* how they should manage sleep. As with so many other aspects of medical complexity, parents are the experts on their children. Conversations about sleep, or any other part of the child's care, needs to keep this truth front and centre.

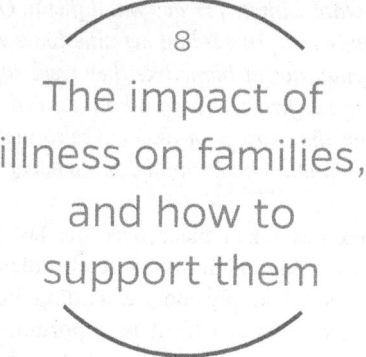

8

The impact of illness on families, and how to support them

In Chapter 1, we reviewed some of the impacts of childhood illness on parents, but we need to consider the impact on the child themselves, as well as their siblings, and grandparents. There are significant practical factors that need to be considered to help families cope, and understanding the pertinent issues will help you to target solutions.

The impact on sick children

Chronic pain in childhood has many impacts on child psychology, and physical wellbeing (Murray et al., 2020) as well as on education, and social and emotional needs (Lum et al., 2019). While children are increasingly living with illness, rather than dying from illness, this also means that children are now living with an illness for a longer period of time, with associated impacts on their physical, mental, and emotional health and wellbeing.

'Hospital life was hard, adjusting to becoming a new

> *mum in a ward with no privacy was difficult. One thing I struggled with accepting is that her milestones were being hit in hospital, not at home like they were supposed to be. She said her first words in a hospital bed, she stood up alone on the ward floor and she celebrated her first Christmas without all our family.'* Roisin Butler

A lot of work has taken place over the last few years to support quality of life in children with chronic illness – after all, healthcare is not simply about extending life, but helping people to thrive. This is why it is important and relevant that early-life conditions are associated with longer-term outcomes, such as adult experiences of pain and depression (Goosby, 2013).

As children move into adolescence, their thoughts and behaviours can become increasingly affected by their health and pain status. One study found that adolescents with chronic pain felt that disability and health anxiety had a negative impact on their sense of independence, and depressed mood and family dysfunction negatively affected their sense of self-identity and emotional adjustment. However, the same adolescents felt that they had better problem-solving skills than their healthy peers. This makes sense, as children with chronic health problems increasingly have to take responsibility for their own health and healthcare. One factor that seemed to buffer the adolescents from some of these negative impacts is peer support – having strong social networks was protective against some of the perceived negative outcomes (Eccleston et al., 2008).

There are five developmental milestones used in research to describe the successful transition from adolescence to adulthood. These are leaving school, starting a career, leaving home, marrying, and becoming a parent. Some more recent research adds psychological maturity to that list (Settersten and Ray, 2010). One could argue that many of these may be irrelevant even for healthy children – for example, young adults may not leave home due to the lack of affordable housing and may choose not to marry or have children. Nevertheless, these milestones remain common in a general sense, and can be useful markers of readiness to leave adolescence behind and develop an adult identity (Kirkpatrick Johnson et al., 2007).

A meta-analysis which included data from nearly 90,000 individuals found that adolescents with chronic illness are less likely to finish education, find employment, leave the parental home, get married and become parents. They also tend to have lower income levels (Pinquart, 2014). These outcomes may be related to differences in functional ability, long periods of absence from school or work, and lack of social opportunities due to long-term illness, and they are also exacerbated in people who have a neurological illness such as epilepsy and cerebral palsy, and sensory impairment such as blindness and deafness – suggesting that these children could benefit from early targeted intervention to improve their access to school and social experiences, as well as adaptations to their environment to reduce the disabling nature of certain places and spaces. There is also clear work to be done on actively addressing and reducing discrimination, for example, offering resources, skills training, and interventions to assist with finding employment and achieving independence (Verhoef et al., 2013).

Siblings

While much of the focus of childhood illness is necessarily on the child, and often the parent who is an ever-present feature of the child's attendance at appointments, what about siblings? Any siblings may be less immediately obvious, and while a social history is always taken in hospital, which accounts for who is present at home and how they may be affected, the needs of siblings may only be acknowledged, rather than actively addressed. Much of the literature related to siblings focuses on childhood cancer, but given that cancer is not a homogenous disease and can affect any body system, for variable lengths of time, the research on this population group may apply to other families.

In a systematic review of the impacts of paediatric intensive care admission, many parents reported spending less time with their healthy children, which caused a strain on the relationship (Abela et al., 2020). This disparity may partly explain the tendency for siblings to experience anger and jealousy (Woodgate, 2006) and other negative impacts on their emotional quality of life (Bravo et al., 2020). Another study found that siblings of children with cancer noted that their family felt 'ripped apart', and there was a shift in the functioning and dynamic of their family – in that the usual roles fulfilled by certain family members changed (Van Schoors et al., 2019), and these changes in personal life were difficult to adapt to (Havill et al., 2019). Healthy siblings report feelings of worry for their ill sibling, as well as sadness, and post-traumatic stress disorder (Long et al., 2015).

> 'Over the period of a year, one of our twin daughters had several admissions to hospital. In fact in that year, she spent 20 weeks in a variety of hospitals, including two unplanned intensive care stays. This had a huge impact not only on our direct family unit, but on extended family as well.
>
> She was a year old when she started to become ill; and almost three years old when most of her symptoms

The impact of illness on families

disappeared. Her illness meant that I couldn't go back to work after my maternity leave, as no employer can reasonably give someone 20 weeks of leave a year, often at very short notice; so we were financially worse off as we lost a full-time wage.

My husband's mental health suffered, as he was expected to continue working (as the only wage earner in the family) as if he didn't have a very ill child at home. His work involved travel abroad, and he often only found out that our daughter was in hospital when he woke up, due to time zone differences. While his employer was great and allowed him time off, he was always very conscious that he needed to continue to work to support the family.

Her hospital admissions got longer as the illness worsened, including a six-week stay in our local hospital. As she got progressively more unwell, we ended up in hospitals further from home. I remember arriving at a hospital 100 miles from our home, at 3am, in a paediatric ambulance with my daughter, who had been put into a medically induced coma, and I had nothing with me except for my purse and a changing bag. Luckily, there was parent accommodation attached to the hospital, but I spent the first 48 hours when my daughter was in intensive care trying to find someone who could drive me somewhere to buy clothes, a toothbrush etc.

Our other twin girl also suffered when her sister was ill. Her Mummy, twin sister and routine disappeared, and she had to be looked after by various relatives in different locations, often being driven to the other side of the country to see me for an hour or so; before being taken to a hotel, or a relative's house. I wasn't able to have both girls on the ward overnight at our local hospital, and siblings aren't allowed onto intensive care units;

so she wasn't able to be with me. Her sister and I often disappeared in the middle of the night, and sometimes she then didn't see me for a week at a time. She has since been diagnosed with anxiety, probably as a direct result of that time.' Shelley Watson

These emotional and psychological impacts are clearly not limited to cancer, despite the plethora of research on this topic. A recent meta-analysis explored the impacts of having an autistic sibling, and found that non-autistic siblings have more behaviour problems, negative beliefs, psychological problems and poorer sibling relationships (Shivers et al., 2019).

While it is obvious that a child with chronic illness would experience absence from school, some studies find that siblings also have higher rates of absence, partly driven by a desire to be with their sick sibling in hospital, which then drives poorer academic functioning (Alderfer et al., 2009). Another study noted that even when at school, siblings are often distracted by thoughts and worries about their sick sibling, and simultaneously find it frustrating to be constantly asked by teachers and peers about their sibling (Prchal and Landolt, 2012).

Chronic ill health can be considered an adverse childhood experience (ACE) for the unwell child, but so too is the loss of a sibling in childhood. Bereavement in childhood is associated with poorer developmental outcomes including future relationships, academic attainment, and career functioning, as well as mental health (Burns et al., 2020). In terms of palliative care, while siblings sometimes report anger and distress when parents give more attention to their dying sibling, the provision of home-based palliative care was protective, as it allowed family functioning to be less disrupted and usual routines could continue to a greater extent – including maintaining contact with extended family, friends, and school (Winger et al., 2020).

> *'The trauma on my older child when my youngest was hospitalised for extended periods of time was one of the hardest things about this experience. Parents need to be aware of the possibility of attachment injury in their other children. We spent extensive time in play therapy and rebuilding familial relationships.'* Brittney Piper

However, notwithstanding the heavy load that siblings of sick children carry, the impacts are not *all* negative – siblings also experience higher social competence and maturity, more compassion and stronger sibling bonds (Yang et al., 2016). Furthermore, the experience of childhood illness often brings families closer together as they work to solve problems, which can also boost resilience (Van Schoors et al., 2019).

Given all the potential negative impacts on siblings, how can those involved in the care of healthy siblings best offer support? The following are suggestions based on current literature and clinical experience:

- Try to avoid making the healthy sibling the disseminator of information. Teachers, family members and others should not ask the healthy sibling for updates. Instead, delegate the task of creating a private blog or newsletter to keep people informed. Some people use social media for this – which has pros and cons. It is obviously easy to update quickly, but also creates a digital footprint about a child, containing deeply personal information.
- Be proactive in telling a child's teachers or carers what is going on so they can be alert to changes in the child's

behaviour, attention, or emotional regulation.
- Talk to the child about topics unrelated to illness. While children should be encouraged to ask whatever questions they want, and volunteer information, this should be on their terms. We should not assume they want to talk about their sick sibling.
- Some research has found that the sights and sounds of PICU, as well as witnessing invasive procedures, can be frightening and traumatic. Parents could consider preparing their child in advance for the environment of PICU – perhaps by showing them images of generic intensive care units on the internet, or recording a video of the machinery to capture the sounds of the equipment. They could also consider whether it would be best to remove their healthy child from the unit if their sibling is about to have an invasive procedure.
- Children will often invent a more frightening reality in their mind if they are not given answers to the questions they ask. Sometimes children ask deeply uncomfortable questions, such as 'will [my sibling] die?'. If we do not provide an answer that they can understand, they are likely to imagine the worst, and may also harbour other irrational fears – such as believing that because their sibling is unwell, that they will also become unwell.
- Help siblings to be involved with caring. Healthy siblings can talk, read, or sing to their sick sibling. They can brush their hair, massage their hands or feet, or help pick out clothes or toys for them.
- Remember to spend one-to-one time with siblings to avoid them feeling like they are less important than the sick child, and as hard as this is, try to make these times about the healthy child and their interests.
- Most healthy children also appreciate nurses and doctors

talking to them. It can be hard to watch so many 'important' people making a fuss over their sibling.
- Refer siblings to psychological support if required. There are different services available, including play therapy, music therapy, art therapy and talking therapies – nothing works in the same way for everyone, but most children benefit from an opportunity to have someone focus on them for a change. I remember my healthy daughter receiving some music therapy and afterwards, she reflected that it was not perhaps the therapy that helped, but more specifically the fact that, for once, her sister had been the one to sit outside in the corridor waiting for the appointment to finish!

It is certainly not inevitable that healthy children will experience negative outcomes from the experience of their sibling being unwell, but it is important to acknowledge this as a risk, to put protective strategies in place, and help the sibling access the support they need.

Grandparents

While not all families have close, integrated relationships with grandparents, the child-grandparent relationship is significant for many. While the influence of grandparents has been found to be interfering, unhelpful, or non-existent in some contexts, grandparents may provide help with childcare, discipline, play, feeding, providing financial assistance, and providing advice and companionship – all of which can support parenting confidence and resilience (Sadruddin et al., 2019). One study found that grandparents needed and wanted to be involved when their grandchild was sick in hospital so that they could support *their* child, as well as their grandchild (Dias and Mendes-Castillo, 2021).

The emotional and psychological needs of bereaved

grandparents have also been the subject of study. Grandparents mourn not only for their grandchild, but also for their grieving adult child, and feel a huge psychological burden to provide support, while managing their own grief (Flury et al., 2021). One study referred to the multi-generational emotional pain of witnessing the grief of their child, surviving grandchildren, and the wider family, as well as their own pain following the death of a child with a life-limiting condition (Tatterton and Walshe, 2019).

On the flip side, the absence of involvement by grandparents may be an additional source of pain, loss and distress to families who have more dysfunctional relationships, or when grandparents are no longer alive or healthy enough to offer this supportive role (Novak-Pavlik et al., 2022). For these families, there may be complex layers of disappointment, hurt and anger, in addition to the stress of having a sick child.

> *'I don't have a close relationship with my mother, and she has remained relatively uninvolved with my children – something I find painful at the best of times. But when my eldest son needed emergency surgery, I called her to ask for help managing the other children and she told me she was too busy. Of course, it was stressful enough having a sick child, but feeling like my own mother didn't care only added to the difficulty.'* Davina Grey

Clearly families and family relationships are complex, and not everyone has the same stressors or sources of support. Some areas to help you consider what support systems already exist and what might be needed include:

- What does the family look like? Is there one parent or are there two?

The impact of illness on families

- Are there any other close family members who are helpful or supportive?
- Are there any siblings, and if so, how are they being affected right now?
- Are there any pets that need to be cared for?
- Does this family need further financial assistance?
- Are there practical supportive measures needed?
- Does the family have any community support?
- What are the usual coping strategies, and can these be utilised?
- Is there an impact on employment, and if so, is there anything that can be done?
- Does the parent have social support, including people who will visit?
- Is respite support needed or appropriate?
- Is a further referral required?

The final section of this book will explore some of these practical approaches to supporting families with sick children. If you are the parent of a sick child, you might find it helpful to put a bookmark here and pass this book to those that support you so they know how best to help you.

How to support families of sick children

Exactly how and to what extent you are involved with supporting a family will depend on the nature of the illness, but also the relationship you have with the family. For some, awareness is all that is needed, whereas for others, you may be intimately involved.

Some of the key ways to help include:

Practical: many families find it hard to think of what they need in a crisis. Rather than asking them if there is anything they need, offer specific help with tasks. If you are not able to do this, suggest that someone close to the family take on this responsibility. A list can be circulated, or a rota, and one person can coordinate who has the front-door key. Common areas of stress that a family might appreciate help with are:

- Food – offering meals is enormously helpful, and not just while in hospital. Not having to plan, shop for and cook nutritious meals takes a huge burden from a family.
- Pets – a common source of guilt and stress is not being able to properly care for a family pet. Offering to clean out the guinea pigs, walk the dog, or feed the cat while a family is resident in hospital eases this mental load.
- Laundry – during prolonged or recurrent admissions, it is hard to keep clothes clean. Not only is there often not a washing machine (or means to dry clothes) in hospital, but the washing at home continues to pile up too if the rest of the family are still at home.
- Housework – all too frequently, families dash to hospital leaving the dirty plates in the sink, and the home needing some TLC. Arriving home to a house that has seen the business end of a vacuum cleaner is a lot less stressful.

Financial: there may be additional benefits or financial supports that families can access. Hospitals will often subsidise parking, but this may not run to travel costs and the costs of existing in hospital. If there is someone who can look up access to financial support this can be a huge help. Some childhood illnesses are covered by adult critical illness cover on life insurance policies, which is one possible avenue to explore, and some charities will provide a one-off grant at the time of diagnosis. A hospital social worker, health visitor or specialist nurse will usually know about access to financial assistance as well.

Logistical: getting people and things from A to B can be hard, and this is one way to help a family under pressure. Offering to do school drop-offs or pick-ups, have siblings over after school, or take care of organising the school or nursery admin might be one option. Another helpful intervention is for someone to give a parent and child a lift to and from hospital – this avoids the need to find and pay for parking and means a stressed parent can just focus on their child, rather than having to drive.

Work: parents of sick children may need to adapt working patterns. Is it possible for them to continue working if they have different hours or a more flexible working policy? Could they do their work if they had certain equipment that they could take to hospital? Or is someone able to sit with the child while the parent goes to work on reduced hours to maintain their source of income? Not all parents will want this option, preferring to stay with their child, but this might be important for longer-term illness.

Social/relational: parents of sick hospitalised children often report isolation, loneliness, and stress. Sometimes they may appreciate company in hospital, and a chance to connect with important people. They may also experience isolation if their child has complex needs and they find it difficult to leave them. In these cases, could someone sit with the child while the parent meets a friend?

Respite: parents of sick children also have reduced opportunities for time away from home, eating out, breaks away or exercise. Having a trusted network of people may mean the difference between being forced to stay at home much of the time, and the confidence to go out.

Optimising wellness more widely

Another aspect to consider is optimising the other aspects of wellness to reduce the likelihood of further illness complications. Social injustices, health inequalities, inequitable access to services or healthcare, and health disparities still exist among many different populations who are variously under-represented, marginalised, oppressed, or stigmatised. Improving health outcomes of chronically unwell children, and reducing the likelihood of long-term impacts and negative outcomes for other family members, involves addressing some of these barriers to health, many of which are institutional (Büyüm et al., 2020). This may be through public health interventions, identifying inequitable access, and challenging practice, as well as advocacy (Nutbeam and Lloyd, 2021). One recent systematic review found that, unfortunately, Black patients are less likely to access timely mental health support due to stigma and mistrust, leading to poorer outcomes. Understanding the cultural and spiritual beliefs of individual cultures, rather than amalgamating all 'non-white' racial groups, would lead to more culturally safe care that meets the needs of specific cultures. Additionally, moving outside of traditional hospital systems and involving community-led groups who understand the culture could address some of these barriers and provide advocacy (Devonport et al., 2023).

Another major barrier to wellness and optimal management of healthcare conditions is lower socioeconomic status, which is a known risk factor for adverse childhood experiences and poorer long-term health outcomes. A recent study did not find that higher socio-economic status buffered a child from the negative consequences of adverse childhood experiences per se; rather lower socio-economic status was associated with more adverse childhood experiences (Houtepen et al., 2020).

Early life experiences are known to shape the central nervous system, cardiovascular system and metabolic health (Haas, 2008; Cohen et al., 2010). Therefore, the stressors a child is exposed to may place them at higher risk for certain poorer health outcomes – which is particularly significant when considering children who may be immunocompromised or medically vulnerable.

Health disparities, reducing the complexity of healthcare, and healthcare provisions are well beyond the scope of this book to address comprehensively, but it would be inappropriate to fail to acknowledge the significant impact of disadvantage and disparities in service provision when discussing some of the public health implications of chronic illness. However, some of the factors that may be more within the control of individuals looking to support families include:

- Optimising diet, including eating foods that are as close to their natural source as possible, plenty of fruits and vegetables, fibre, and wholegrains. Processed foods frequently lack fibre and are high in sugar and trans fats, which are associated with poorer health outcomes (Khandpur et al., 2020). This is where others can really help, because not only are these foods more expensive (further adding to inequalities), but they take more time to cook from scratch as well – which may simply be unachievable for families with sick children.
- Promote physical activity if possible. Although some children have restricted mobility or very complex health needs which limit capacity to exercise, those who can, should avoid sedentary behaviour and exercise within their capability, as this is known to promote better physical and mental health (Chaput et al., 2020). For children with limited mobility, a physiotherapist will be able to provide

some exercises that are possible, and getting outside can really help as well.
- Build parenting self-efficacy, which has been shown to reduce stress and optimise diabetic control among children with type 1 diabetes (Bassi et al., 2021).
- Teach parents about stress management, goal setting, challenging negative self-talk, and making memories, as this has been found to build resilience and decrease stress (Rosenberg et al., 2019).
- Provide parenting support focused on authoritative parenting, as this is associated with better psychosocial adjustment to chronic illness despite reduced family resilience. Authoritative parenting is characterised by a high warmth, low criticism style of parenting, with age-appropriate boundaries (Qiu et al., 2021).

How hospitals can get better

There is plenty that supporters, families, and individuals can do to support parents during childhood illness. But what about hospitals? What interventions do families find supportive and how can they do better? I genuinely believe that one of the most helpful approaches to paediatric clinical care is full adoption of individualised family-centred care. A model that values parents as partners, and is willing to be flexible about certain protocols and policies, can reduce stress for families.

'Our hospital was very supportive in that it let me share a bed with my breastfeeding baby who was receiving chemo. Though I realise not every circumstance would allow for this, it was meaningful to have the hospital acknowledge the importance of the continued routine and bond for my baby and give us the ability to continue something we had been doing at home in a safe way. I

The impact of illness on families

appreciated that in many areas our hospital was flexible and strived to work towards accepting diverse familial and cultural practices.' Brittney Piper

Many parents also want better practical facilities, including beds, food, flexible visiting policies, financial assistance, and laundry facilities.

'We have had our fair share of experiences in hospital. It is hard enough as a parent to see your child unwell enough to be in hospital and it is a pity that there are so many practical challenges that only add to your stress during that time.

I would love to see families in hospital supported better in terms of facilities to stay overnight. I have never had anything other than an incredibly uncomfortable chair to sleep in which means that I barely sleep during the entire admission. Added to that is that we cosleep at home which has never been facilitated in hospital – because Reuben is two, they have always insisted he has a cot and not a bed I could share, which means he sleeps all night on top of me in the uncomfortable chair instead.

Other practical things that we have at times had access to (but not always) have been a 'parent kitchen' with facilities to store and heat food, make a cup of tea etc. Not having this means spending a lot of money on food and coffee (any parent in hospital knows this is essential) on top of travel, car parking and then loss of earnings, it all adds to the financial stress.

Something that I think is a new challenge since the pandemic is that only one parent is allowed on the ward at a time when we have been admitted. Reuben is always very distressed by even coming in the front doors of the

hospital as it is so familiar to him now. I never leave him alone when he is admitted because I know he would be distressed, so if he can't leave the room because he needs oxygen or IV medication then I simply won't eat, drink, or use the bathroom for prolonged periods of time. At least providing parents with meals would help to solve part of that problem and just being compassionate, acknowledging why I wouldn't want to leave him to attend to my own needs and offer to stay with him for five minutes if my partner isn't allowed to be there rather than suggest "he'll be fine". Gemma Nixon

Finally, communicating information with parents should be honest, individualised, compassionate, humble, culturally safe and strengths-based:

Honest: letting parents know what information there is to know, without withholding key details. Parents do not want information sugar-coated, but they want to know the truth, even if it is difficult. We should also let parents know what we do *not* know.

Individualised: I mean this in two ways. Firstly, that acknowledgement should be made of the individual nature of the response to a condition or diagnosis. All children are different, even with the same illness. Secondly, that information-sharing should be tailored to the needs of the family. Do they have the capacity to hear and understand right now? Do they need to hear information in small chunks to allow them to digest it? Do they need someone with them as they hear a diagnosis?

Compassionate: most healthcare professionals are kind, but it is always worth a reminder that even when a clinician has dealt with 1,000 cases of the same condition, they should never become desensitised to how huge and scary this diagnosis might feel to a parent. While it is unhelpful for clinicians to fall apart while delivering a diagnosis, it helps a family to know that the clinician cares about their child.

Humble: clinicians should readily acknowledge what they do not know. It is not a sign of incompetence to own the gaps in their knowledge – particularly when they relate to the child's individual manifestation of their condition, or when it is a rare condition about which there is little prior knowledge.

Culturally safe: many parents are affected by their own anxieties and mistrust of hospital institutions and people in positions of power. This is made worse when professionals do not understand the cultural diversity of families, or when there is a language barrier. Adopting a respectful approach and breaking down hierarchical barriers when caring for families who do not share the culture of the professional may help the family to feel less stressed and anxious.

Strengths-based: no child should be defined by their condition or illness. While parenting through childhood illness may be difficult or different from caring for healthy or typically developing children, most parents would rather focus on their child's many positive attributes.

Validating the experience and paying it forward

Many parents develop strength and resilience through childhood illness and while they would not necessarily say they are grateful for their child's illness or medical complexity, for many families the experience can become a source of strength. Consequently, many families choose to both validate and celebrate their experiences – either by fundraising, advocacy work or raising awareness. Some like to mark their child's strength in art, photography, creativity, something beautiful, nature, or a tangible memento of their experience. Some parents choose to support other families going through similar experiences.

> 'Looking back on our journey so far, I seek comfort in supporting other families going through a new diagnosis and treatment. The power of social media has connected me with so many wonderful people that are walking a similar path to ours.
>
> Someone told me once that you are allowed to accept those feelings of anger and sadness, have those emotions, and let yourself cry. You need them but you also need the days where you laugh until you cry with your child, the nurses, or other families. You will develop strength like you have never known before, not because you want to but because you had to. That strength comes from the pride you feel seeing your child fighting the most difficult battle but still filling your days with smiles. I am strong because of my daughter.' Roisin Butler

Conclusion

Childhood illness is common, and increasingly, children with complex health needs are being supported to live and thrive at home. It was Ambassador Matthew Rycroft of the UK Mission to the UN who said:

> 'How a society treats its most vulnerable is always the measure of its humanity.'

This couldn't be more applicable to this population, and in practice it means that as childhood illness becomes something that more people are supporting, there is more need to develop services for families that do not merely focus on surviving, but thriving.

Childhood illness is not easy – not for the children, families, communities, or healthcare systems. But we owe it to children and families to open-mindedly consider how we can develop best practice. Sometimes this is uncomfortable, inconvenient, or requires a shift in thinking, and this can be hard for those who are used to delivering expert care. But in coming round to a family-centred, individualised and compassionate approach to care, professionals need to accept the truth that families really are the experts on their children.

Part of this shift in thinking is adopting a strengths-based, positive approach to illness and disability. This can be hard to balance alongside an understanding and compassion for those who have life-limiting conditions or whose care has shifted to a palliative approach. But I have never met a bereaved parent who regretted embracing their child's strengths and brilliance. I have never met the parent of a medically complex child who wouldn't rather focus on their child's sense of humour, smile, perseverance, or character. However hard illness can be, and however cruel the prognosis, being positive and encouraging about a child's potential and their unique place in their family is always appropriate.

> 'Real superheroes live in the hearts of small children fighting big battles.' Anon

Resources

If you are caring for or involved with a child with a medical condition or disability, you may find it helpful to check out the following resources:

Complex conditions

www.sickchildrenstrust.org
www.bornattherighttime.com
www.colabpartnership.org.uk

Parental well-being

Being the parent of a sick or medically complex child can be challenging. Parents need to remember to take care of themselves. Here are some resources to help:

Self-care activities: formeasaparent.com/the-intervention-tools/self-care-activities and at parentselfcare.com and www.psychologytoday.com/us/blog/joyful-parenting/201708/25-simple-self-care-tools-parents. Headspace and Calm are good apps as well. Beadsofcourageuk.org are a charity who provide a coloured bead to represent various procedures that children undergo to tangibly show their strength.

Financial and practical support

If parents have life insurance with critical illness cover, it is worth checking to see if they can make a claim on their insurance. This often applies even though the child is not named on the policy and will have no effect on their own cover. Please also check with the social worker, or medical team.

www.moneyadviceservice.org.uk/en/articles/financial-support-if-you-or-your-child-has-a-disability
www.familyfund.org.uk/
www.gov.uk/disability-living-allowance-children

UK-based support regarding government aided support: www.gov.uk/browse/childcare-parenting/financial-help-children

Also check with the hospital – they may have funds and grants to assist with parking, accommodation, and some charities provide a one-off grant.

Accommodation may be provided by the hospital, or there may be a home-from-home organisation near the hospital, if a child is cared for far from home. Try Ronald McDonald house: rmhc.org.uk

If friends ask what they can do to help, a meal train can take the hassle out of coordinating meals: www.mealtrain.com

Pregnancy and birth

If a mother or parent is pregnant and wants to find out more about their options in labour and birth, in the first case they can ask their midwife or obstetrician. If the child is diagnosed with a condition antenatally, they will probably be offered the opportunity to look around the neonatal unit. If not – please ask.

www.bliss.org.uk/parents/about-your-baby/before-birth
www.birthrights.org.uk
www.wrisk.org
www.arc-uk.org
www.infantrisk.com

Resources

Feeding support

Some information here about using a nasogastric (NG) tube: www.gosh.nhs.uk/teenagers/your-condition/tests-and-treatments/nasogastric-ng-tube-feeding

The Breastfeeding the Brave Facebook group is here: www.facebook.com/groups/358557901478129

First Steps Nutrition Trust – unbiased information about formula, including specialised formula: www.firststepsnutrition.org

Some information about using a gastrostomy (G tube):

www.cps.ca/en/documents/position/gastrostomy-tube-feeding

www.feedingtubeawareness.org/g-tube

www.gosh.nhs.uk/conditions-and-treatments/procedures-and-treatments/living-gastrostomy-feeding-device

www.feedingmatters.org

Acknowledgements

I must firstly thank the hundreds of families I have had the honour of supporting over the years. They have witnessed my many mistakes as I have grown and learned from them, and they have been gracious and patient when I have got it wrong. I am also indebted to the many parents I have had the privilege of interviewing for my research, and the numerous parents who contributed quotes and meaningful segments for this book. Their courage and strength astound me.

Secondly, I need to honour the hundreds of dedicated paediatric healthcare professionals who have inspired, taught, and mentored me. I am more grateful than I can say that there are so many incredible clinicians caring for families in paediatrics – believe me, there are *many* people who care about all the issues in this book (as well as the ones I couldn't do justice to). Writing about healthcare improvements is hard when I know full well that every day, stalwart and stoical professionals show up and deliver exemplary care as standard, albeit within a system that sometimes feels stretched to breaking point. All of us can grow and improve, but none of that can happen without a genuine love for their job, which they have in spades.

Thirdly, thank you to the team at Pinter & Martin for seeing the value in this topic, for their support, and welcoming childhood illness into the *Why It Matters* collection.

Finally, I must once again thank my family, particularly my children, who have endured more than their fair share of illness and family upheaval due to illness. They were the ones who taught me that bravery is not the absence of fear, but the grit and determination to see the fear and keep going anyway. Turns out, childhood illness can take many things away, but it cannot crush your spirit.

References

Introduction

Kanthimathinathan, H. K., Plunkett, A., Scholefield, B. R., Pearson, G. A., & Morris, K. P. (2020). Trends in long-stay admissions to a UK paediatric intensive care unit. *Archives of Disease in Childhood*, 105(6), 558-562.

Keeble, E., & Kossarova, L. (2017). Focus on: Emergency hospital care for children and young people. Focus On Research Report. Quality Watch.

Chapter 1

Compas, B. E., Jaser, S. S., Dunn, M. J., & Rodriguez, E. M. (2012). Coping with chronic illness in childhood and adolescence. *Annual Review of Clinical Psychology*, 8, 455-480.

Dominguez, S. K., Matthijssen, S. J., & Lee, C. W. (2021). Trauma-focused treatments for depression. A systematic review and meta-analysis. *PLoS One*, 16(7), e0254778.

Foster, K., Young, A., Mitchell, R., Van, C., & Curtis, K. (2017). Experiences and needs of parents of critically injured children during the acute hospital phase: a qualitative investigation. *Injury*, 48(1), 114-120.

Franck, L. S., Wray, J., Gay, C., Dearmun, A. K., Lee, K., & Cooper, B. A. (2015). Predictors of parent post-traumatic stress symptoms after child hospitalization on general pediatric wards: a prospective cohort study. *International Journal of Nursing Studies*, 52(1), 10-21.

Gannoni, A. F., & Shute, R. H. (2010). Parental and child perspectives on adaptation to childhood chronic illness: A qualitative study. *Clinical Child Psychology and Psychiatry*, 15(1), 39-53.

Law, E., Fisher, E., Eccleston, C., & Palermo, T. M. (2019). Psychological interventions for parents of children and adolescents with chronic illness. *Cochrane Database of Systematic Reviews*, (3).

McIlroy, P. A., King, R. S., Garrouste-Orgeas, M., Tabah, A., & Ramanan, M. (2019). The effect of ICU diaries on psychological outcomes and quality of life of survivors of critical illness and their relatives: a systematic review and meta-analysis. *Critical Care Medicine*, 47(2), 273-279.

Mortensen, J., Simonsen, B. O., Eriksen, S. B., Skovby, P., Dall, R., & Elklit, A. (2015). Family-centred care and traumatic symptoms in parents of children admitted to PICU. *Scandinavian Journal of Caring Sciences*, 29(3), 495-500.

Muscara, F., McCarthy, M. C., Woolf, C., Hearps, S. J. C., Burke, K., & Anderson, V. A. (2015). Early psychological reactions in parents of children with a life threatening illness within a pediatric hospital setting. *European Psychiatry*, 30(5), 555-561.

Pelentsov, L. J., Laws, T. A., & Esterman, A. J. (2015). The supportive care needs of parents caring for a child with a rare disease: a scoping review. *Disability and Health Journal*, 8(4), 475-491.

Pinquart, M. (2013). Do the parent–child relationship and parenting behaviors differ between families with a child with and without chronic illness? A meta-analysis. *Journal of Pediatric Psychology*, 38(7), 708-721.

Rodriguez, E. M., Dunn, M. J., Zuckerman, T., Vannatta, K., Gerhardt, C. A., & Compas, B. E. (2012). Cancer-related sources of stress for children with cancer and their parents. *Journal of Pediatric Psychology*, 37(2), 185-197.

Smith, J., Cheater, F., & Bekker, H. (2015). Parents' experiences of living with a child with a long-term condition: a rapid structured review of the literature. *Health Expectations*, 18(4), 452-474.

Woolf, C., Muscara, F., Anderson, V. A., & McCarthy, M. C. (2016). Early traumatic stress responses in parents following a serious illness in their child: A systematic review. *Journal of Clinical Psychology in Medical Settings*, 23(1), 53-66.

Chapter 3

Hookway, L., Brown, A., & Grant, A. (2023). Breastfeeding sick children in hospital: Exploring the experiences of mothers in UK paediatric wards. *Maternal & Child Nutrition*, 19(2), e13489.

Lambert, V., Matthews, A., MacDonell, R., & Fitzsimons, J. (2017). Paediatric early warning systems for detecting and responding to clinical deterioration in children: a systematic review. *BMJ Open*, 7(3), e014497.

Manocha, S., & Taneja, N. (2016). Assessment of paediatric pain: a critical review. *Journal of Basic and Clinical Physiology and Pharmacology*, 27(4), 323-331.

Perasso, G., Camurati, G., Morrin, E., Dill, C., Dolidze, K., Clegg, T., ... & Rippen, H. (2021). Five reasons why pediatric settings should integrate the play specialist and five issues in practice. *Frontiers in Psychology*, 12, 687292.

Chapter 4

Ainsworth, M. S. (1979). Infant–mother attachment. *American Psychologist*, 34(10), 932.

Ainsworth, M. D. (1962). The effects of maternal deprivation: A review of findings and controversy in the context of research strategy. *Public Health Papers*, 14, 97-165.

Ames, K. E., Rennick, J. E., & Baillargeon, S. (2011). A qualitative interpretive study exploring parents' perception of the parental role in the paediatric intensive care unit. *Intensive and Critical Care Nursing*, 27(3), 143-150.

Beck, A. F., Solan, L. G., Brunswick, S. A., Sauers-Ford, H., Simmons, J. M., Shah, S., ... & H2O Study Group. (2017). Socioeconomic status influences the toll paediatric hospitalisations take on families: a qualitative study. *BMJ Qual Saf*, 26(4), 304-311.

Bélanger, L., Bussières, S., Rainville, F., Coulombe, M., & Desmartis, M. (2017). Hospital visiting policies–impacts on patients, families and staff: a review of the literature to inform decision making. *Journal of Hospital Administration*, 6(6), 51-62.

Bowlby, J. (1969). Attachment and loss, Vol. 1.(pp.) Attachment. NY: Basic Books.

Brazelton, T. (1974). The origins of reciprocity: The early mother-infant interaction. The effect of the infant on its caregiver, 49-76.

Butler, A., Copnell, B., & Willetts, G. (2014). Family-centred care in the paediatric intensive care unit: an integrative review of the literature. *Journal of Clinical*

References

Nursing, 23(15-16), 2086-2100.

Central Health Services Council (Great Britain). Committee on the Welfare of Children in Hospital, & Platt, S. H. (1959). *The welfare of children in hospital*. HM Stationery Office.

Harlow, H. F. (1958). The nature of love. *American Psychologist*, 13(12), 673.

Hill, C., Knafl, K. A., Docherty, S., & Santacroce, S. J. (2019). Parent perceptions of the impact of the Paediatric Intensive Care environment on delivery of family-centred care. *Intensive and Critical Care Nursing*, 50, 88-94.

Ivany, A., LeBlanc, C., Grisdale, M., Maxwell, B., & Langley, J. M. (2016). Reducing infection transmission in the playroom: Balancing patient safety and family-centered care. *American Journal of Infection Control*, 44(1), 61-65.

Kish, A. M., Newcombe, P. A., & Haslam, D. M. (2018). Working and caring for a child with chronic illness: a review of current literature. *Child: Care, Health and Development*, 44(3), 343-354.

Nielsen, J. S., Agbeko, R., Bate, J., Jordan, I., Dohna-Schwake, C., Potratz, J., ... & Wösten-van Asperen, R. M. (2022). Organizational characteristics of European pediatric onco-critical care: An international cross-sectional survey. *Frontiers in Pediatrics*, 10, 1024273.

Nimmo, S. (2019). Please don't call me mum. *BMJ*, 367.

Prescott, J. W. (1975). Body pleasure and the origins of violence. *Bulletin of the Atomic Scientists*, 31(9), 10-20.

Rempel, G. R., Ravindran, V., Rogers, L. G., & Magill-Evans, J. (2013). Parenting under pressure: A grounded theory of parenting young children with life-threatening congenital heart disease. *Journal of Advanced Nursing*, 69(3), 619-630.

Rutter, M. (1987). Psychosocial resilience and protective mechanisms. *American Journal of Orthopsychiatry*, 57(3), 316-331.

Schaeffer, H. R., & Emerson, P. E. (1964). Patterns of response to physical contact in early human development. *Journal of Child Psychology & Psychiatry*.

Schore, J. R., & Schore, A. N. (2008). Modern attachment theory: The central role of affect regulation in development and treatment. *Clinical Social Work Journal*, 36(1), 9-20.

Shields, L. (2015). What is "family-centred care"? *European Journal for Person Centered Healthcare*, 3(2), 139-144.

Thomson, J., Shah, S. S., Simmons, J. M., Sauers-Ford, H. S., Brunswick, S., Hall, D., ... & Beck, A. F. (2016). Financial and social hardships in families of children with medical complexity. *The Journal of Pediatrics*, 172, 187-193.

Van den Hoogen, A., & Ketelaar, M. (2022). Parental involvement and empowerment in paediatric critical care: Partnership is key! *Nursing in Critical Care*, 27(3), 294.

Van der Horst, F. C., & Van der Veer, R. (2008). Loneliness in infancy: Harry Harlow, John Bowlby and issues of separation. *Integrative Psychological and Behavioral Science*, 42, 325-335.

Van Oers, H. A., Haverman, L., Limperg, P. F., van Dijk-Lokkart, E. M., Maurice-Stam, H., & Grootenhuis, M. A. (2014). Anxiety and depression in mothers and fathers of a chronically ill child. *Maternal and Child Health Journal*, 18(8), 1993-2002.

Vonneilich, N., Lüdecke, D., & Kofahl, C. (2016). The impact of care on family and health-related quality of life of parents with chronically ill and disabled children. *Disability and Rehabilitation*, 38(8), 761-767.

Watson, J. B. (1913). Psychology as the behaviorist views it. *Psychological Review*, 20(2), 158.

Chapter 5

Academy of Breastfeeding Medicine. (2012). ABM clinical protocol# 25: recommendations for preprocedural fasting for the breastfed infant: "NPO" guidelines. *Breastfeeding Medicine*, 7(3), 197-202.

Azak, M., Aksucu, G., & Çağlar, S. (2022). The effect of parental Presence on Pain levels of children during invasive procedures: A systematic review. *Pain Management Nursing*, 23(5), 682-688.

Compton, S., Madgy, A., Goldstein, M., Sandhu, J., Dunne, R., & Swor, R. (2006). Emergency medical service providers' experience with family presence during cardiopulmonary resuscitation. *Resuscitation*, 70(2), 223-228.

Dainty, K. N., Atkins, D. L., Breckwoldt, J., Maconochie, I., Schexnayder, S. M., Skrifvars, M. B., ... & Yeung, J. (2021). Family presence during resuscitation in paediatric and neonatal cardiac arrest: A systematic review. *Resuscitation*, 162, 20-34.

De Lourdes Levy, M., Larcher, V., Kurz, R., & members of the Ethics Working Group of the CESP. (2003). Informed consent/assent in children. Statement of the Ethics Working Group of the Confederation of European Specialists in Paediatrics (CESP). *European Journal of Pediatrics*, 162, 629-633.

Frykholm, P., Disma, N., Andersson, H., Beck, C., Bouvet, L., Cercueil, E., ... & Afshari, A. (2022). Pre-operative fasting in children: A guideline from the European Society of Anaesthesiology and Intensive Care. *European Journal of Anaesthesiology*, 39(1), 4-25.

Harrison, D., & Bueno, M. (2023). Translating evidence: pain treatment in newborns, infants, and toddlers during needle-related procedures. *Pain Reports*, 8(2).

Harrison, D., Reszel, J., Bueno, M., Sampson, M., Shah, V. S., Taddio, A., ... & Turner, L. (2016). Breastfeeding for procedural pain in infants beyond the neonatal period. *Cochrane Database of Systematic Reviews*, (10).

Jensen, L., & Kosowan, S. (2011). Family presence during cardiopulmonary resuscitation: cardiac health care professionals' perspectives. *Canadian Journal of Cardiovascular Nursing*, 21(3).

Johnston, C., Campbell-Yeo, M., Disher, T., Benoit, B., Fernandes, A., Streiner, D., ... & Zee, R. (2017). Skin-to-skin care for procedural pain in neonates. *Cochrane Database of Systematic Reviews*, (2).

Matziou, V., Chrysostomou, A., Vlahioti, E., & Perdikaris, P. (2013). Parental presence and distraction during painful childhood procedures. *British Journal of Nursing*, 22(8), 470-475.

McClenathan, C. B. M., Torrington, C. K. G., & Uyehara, C. F. (2002). Family member presence during cardiopulmonary resuscitation: a survey of US and international critical care professionals. *Chest*, 122(6), 2204-2211.

References

Sak-Dankosky, N., Andruszkiewicz, P., Sherwood, P. R., & Kvist, T. (2014). Integrative review: nurses' and physicians' experiences and attitudes towards inpatient-witnessed resuscitation of an adult patient. *Journal of Advanced Nursing*, 70(5), 957-974.

Shah, P. S., Herbozo, C., Aliwalas, L. L., & Shah, V. S. (2012). Breastfeeding or breast milk for procedural pain in neonates. *Cochrane Database of Systematic Reviews*, (12).

Stevens, B., Yamada, J., Ohlsson, A., Haliburton, S., & Shorkey, A. (2016). Sucrose for analgesia in newborn infants undergoing painful procedures. *Cochrane Database of Systematic Reviews*, (7).

Vittinghoff, M., Lönnqvist, P. A., Mossetti, V., Heschl, S., Simic, D., Colovic, V., ... & Morton, N. S. (2018). Postoperative pain management in children: Guidance from the pain committee of the European Society for Paediatric Anaesthesiology (ESPA Pain Management Ladder Initiative). *Pediatric Anesthesia*, 28(6), 493-506.

Yaster, M. (2010). Multimodal analgesia in children. *European Journal of Anaesthiology*, 27(10), 851-857.

Chapter 6

Banks, S. (2022). *Why Formula Feeding Matters*. Pinter & Martin.

Braegger, C., Decsi, T., Dias, J. A., Hartman, C., Kolacek, S., Koletzko, B., ... & ESPGHAN Committee on Nutrition. (2010). Practical approach to paediatric enteral nutrition: a comment by the ESPGHAN committee on nutrition. *Journal of Pediatric Gastroenterology and Nutrition*, 51(1), 110-122.

Brenner, M., O'Shea, M., Clancy, A., Kamionka, S. L., Larkin, P., Lignou, S., ... & Hilliard, C. (2019). Services and Boundary Negotiations for Children with Complex Care Needs in Europe. In Issues and Opportunities in Primary Health Care for Children in Europe: The Final Summarised Results of the Models of Child Health Appraised (MOCHA) Project (pp. 199-218). Emerald Publishing Limited.

Brown, A. (2017). *Why Starting Solids Matters*. Pinter & Martin.

Cohn, L. N., Pechlivanoglou, P., Lee, Y., Mahant, S., Orkin, J., Marson, A., & Cohen, E. (2020). Health outcomes of parents of children with chronic illness: a systematic review and meta-analysis. *The Journal of Pediatrics*, 218, 166-177.

Everitt, L. H., Awoseyila, A., Bhatt, J. M., Johnson, M. J., Vollmer, B., & Evans, H. J. (2021). Weaning oxygen in infants with bronchopulmonary dysplasia. *Paediatric Respiratory Reviews*, 39, 82-89.

Fairfax, A., Brehaut, J., Colman, I., Sikora, L., Kazakova, A., Chakraborty, P., & Potter, B. K. (2019). A systematic review of the association between coping strategies and quality of life among caregivers of children with chronic illness and/or disability. *BMC Pediatrics*, 19(1), 1-16.

Feudtner, C., Nye, R. T., Boyden, J. Y., Schwartz, K. E., Korn, E. R., Dewitt, A. G., ... & Hill, D. L. (2021). Association between children with life-threatening conditions and their parents' and siblings' mental and physical health. *JAMA Network Open*, 4(12), e2137250-e2137250.

Fumarola, S., Allaway, R., Callaghan, R., Collier, M., Downie, F., Geraghty, J., ... & Voegeli, D. (2020). Overlooked and underestimated: medical adhesive-related skin injuries. *Journal of Wound Care*, 29(Sup3c), S1-S24.

Glasson, E. J., Forbes, D., Ravikumara, M., Nagarajan, L., Wilson, A., Jacoby, P., ... & Downs, J. (2020). Gastrostomy and quality of life in children with intellectual disability: a qualitative study. *Archives of Disease in Childhood*, 105(10), 969-974.

Homan, M., Hauser, B., Romano, C., Tzivinikos, C., Torroni, F., Gottrand, F., ... & Amil-Dias, J. (2021). Percutaneous endoscopic gastrostomy in children: an update to the ESPGHAN position paper. *Journal of Pediatric Gastroenterology and Nutrition*, 73(3), 415-426.

Hookway, L. (2022). *Breastfeeding the Brave*. Thought Rebellion.

Järvelä, M., Katila, M., Eskola, V., Mäkinen, R., Mandelin, P., Saarenpää-Heikkilä, O., & Lauhkonen, E. (2023). Paediatric home respiratory support-review of patient selection and when to finish? *ERJ Open Research*, 9: Suppl. 11, 46.

Kazak, A. E., Kassam-Adams, N., Schneider, S., Zelikovsky, N., Alderfer, M. A., & Rourke, M. (2006). An integrative model of pediatric medical traumatic stress. *Journal of Pediatric Psychology*, 31(4), 343-355.

Luzi, D., Pecoraro, F., Tamburis, O., O'Shea, M., Larkin, P., Berry, J., & Brenner, M. (2019). Modelling collaboration of primary and secondary care for children with complex care needs: long-term ventilation as an example. *European Journal of Pediatrics*, 178, 891-901.

Namachivayam, P., Shann, F., Shekerdemian, L., Taylor, A., van Sloten, I., Delzoppo, C., ... & Butt, W. (2010). Three decades of pediatric intensive care: Who was admitted, what happened in intensive care, and what happened afterward. *Pediatric Critical Care Medicine*, 11(5), 549-555.

NICE (2021) cks.nice.org.uk/topics/obstructive-sleep-apnoea-syndrome

Nilsson, S., Ohlen, J., Hessman, E., & Brännström, M. (2020). Paediatric palliative care: a systematic review. *BMJ Supportive & Palliative Care*, 10(2), 157-163.

Oliver, M.(1983). *Social Work with Disabled People*. Basingstoke: Macmillan

Page, B. F., Hinton, L., Harrop, E., & Vincent, C. (2020). The challenges of caring for children who require complex medical care at home: 'The go between for everyone is the parent and as the parent that's an awful lot of responsibility'. *Health Expectations*, 23(5), 1144-1154.

Peat, G., Delaney, S. A., Gibson, F., Fraser, L. K., & Brierley, J. (2023). Shared decision-making experiences in child long-term ventilation: a systematic review. *European Respiratory Review*, 32(169).

Perez Jolles, M., Lengnick-Hall, R., & Mittman, B. S. (2019). Core functions and forms of complex health interventions: a patient-centered medical home illustration. *Journal of General Internal Medicine*, 34, 1032-1038.

Pinquart, M. (2019). Posttraumatic stress symptoms and disorders in parents of children and adolescents with chronic physical illnesses: a meta-analysis. *Journal of Traumatic Stress*, 32(1), 88-96.

Pironi, L., Boeykens, K., Bozzetti, F., Joly, F., Klek, S., Lal, S., ... & Bischoff, S. C. (2020). ESPEN guideline on home parenteral nutrition. *Clinical Nutrition*, 39(6), 1645-1666.

Rennick, J. E., St-Sauveur, I., Knox, A. M., & Ruddy, M. (2019). Exploring the experiences of parent caregivers of children with chronic medical complexity during pediatric intensive care unit hospitalization: an interpretive descriptive study. *BMC Pediatrics*, 19(1), 1-10.

References

Steen, E. H., Wang, X., Boochoon, K. S., Ewing, D. C., Strang, H. E., Kaul, A., ... & Keswani, S. (2020). Wound healing and wound care in neonates: current therapies and novel options. *Advances in Skin & Wound Care*, 33(6), 294-300.

Triantafyllou, C., Chorianopoulou, E., Kourkouni, E., Zaoutis, T. E., & Kourlaba, G. (2021). Prevalence, incidence, length of stay and cost of healthcare-acquired pressure ulcers in pediatric populations: a systematic review and meta-analysis. *International Journal of Nursing Studies*, 115, 103843.

Wallis, C., Paton, J. Y., Beaton, S., & Jardine, E. (2011). Children on long-term ventilatory support: 10 years of progress. *Archives of Disease in Childhood*, 96(11), 998-1002.

Weaver, M. S., Heinze, K. E., Kelly, K. P., Wiener, L., Casey, R. L., Bell, C. J., ... & Hinds, P. S. (2015). Palliative care as a standard of care in pediatric oncology. *Pediatric Blood & Cancer*, 62(S5), S829-S833.

Wong, M., Taylor, E., Longland, R., Leclerc, M., Williams, G., Neylan, M., ... & Chawla, J. (2021). P162 Heated humidified high flow nasal cannula versus continuous positive airway pressure therapy for obstructive sleep apnoea in children: the patients' perspective. *Sleep Advances: A Journal of the Sleep Research Society*, 2(Suppl 1), A74.

Woolf, C., Muscara, F., Anderson, V. A., & McCarthy, M. C. (2016). Early traumatic stress responses in parents following a serious illness in their child: A systematic review. *Journal of Clinical Psychology in Medical Settings*, 23, 53-66.

Wright-Sexton, L. A., Compretta, C. E., Blackshear, C., & Henderson, C. M. (2020). Isolation in parents and providers of children with chronic critical illness. *Pediatric Critical Care Medicine*, 21(8), e530-e537.

Xiao, L., Baker, A., Voutsas, G., Massicotte, C., Wolter, N. E., Propst, E. J., & Narang, I. (2021). Positional device therapy for the treatment of positional obstructive sleep apnea in children: a pilot study. *Sleep Medicine*, 85, 313-316.

Chapter 7

Ball, H. L., Howel, D., Bryant, A., Best, E., Russell, C., & Ward-Platt, M. (2016). Bed-sharing by breastfeeding mothers: who bed-shares and what is the relationship with breastfeeding duration? *Acta Paediatrica*, 105(6), 628-634.

Ball, H. L., Ward-Platt, M. P., Heslop, E., Leech, S. J., & Brown, K. A. (2006). Randomised trial of infant sleep location on the postnatal ward. *Archives of Disease in Childhood*, 91(12), 1005-1010.

Bassi, G., Mancinelli, E., Di Riso, D., & Salcuni, S. (2021). Parental stress, anxiety and depression symptoms associated with self-efficacy in paediatric type 1 diabetes: a literature review. *International Journal of Environmental Research and Public Health*, 18(1), 152.

Blair, P. S., Ball, H. L., McKenna, J. J., Feldman-Winter, L., Marinelli, K. A., Bartick, M. C., & Academy of Breastfeeding Medicine. (2020). Bedsharing and breastfeeding: the academy of breastfeeding medicine protocol# 6, Revision 2019. *Breastfeeding Medicine*, 15(1), 5-16.

Camfferman, D., Kennedy, J. D., Gold, M., Martin, A. J., Winwood, P., & Lushington, K. (2010). Eczema, sleep, and behavior in children. *Journal of Clinical Sleep Medicine*, 6(6), 581-588.

Castro-Rodriguez, J. A., Brockmann, P. E., & Marcus, C. L. (2017). Relation between asthma and sleep disordered breathing in children: is the association causal? *Paediatric Respiratory Reviews*, 22, 72-75.

Dorris, L., Scott, N., Zuberi, S., Gibson, N., & Espie, C. (2008). Sleep problems in children with neurological disorders. *Developmental Neurorehabilitation*, 11(2), 95-114.

Greaves, M. (2006). Infection, immune responses and the aetiology of childhood leukaemia. *Nature Reviews Cancer*, 6(3), 193-203.

Hookway, L. (2021). *Still Awake*. Pinter & Martin.

Hookway, L., Brown, A., & Grant, A. (2023). Breastfeeding sick children in hospital: Exploring the experiences of mothers in UK paediatric wards. *Maternal & Child Nutrition*, 19(2), e13489.

Hulst, R. Y., Gorter, J. W., Voorman, J. M., Kolk, E., Van Der Vossen, S., Visser-Meily, J. M., ... & Verschuren, O. (2021). Sleep problems in children with cerebral palsy and their parents. *Developmental Medicine & Child Neurology*, 63(11), 1344-1350.

Hulst, R. Y., Voorman, J. M., Pillen, S., Ketelaar, M., Visser-Meily, J. M., & Verschuren, O. (2022). Parental perspectives on care for sleep in children with cerebral palsy: a wake-up call. *Disability and Rehabilitation*, 44(3), 458-467.

Hysing, M., Sivertsen, B., Stormark, K. M., Elgen, I., & Lundervold, A. J. (2009). Sleep in children with chronic illness, and the relation to emotional and behavioral problems—a population-based study. *Journal of Pediatric Psychology*, 34(6), 665-670.

Jiménez, E. L., Barrios, R., Calvo, J. C., de la Rosa, M. T., Campillo, J. S., Bayona, J. C., & Bravo, M. (2015). Association of oral breathing with dental malocclusions and general health in children. *Minerva Pediatrica*, 69(3), 188-193.

Kavanagh, J., Jackson, D. J., & Kent, B. D. (2018). Sleep and asthma. *Current Opinion in Pulmonary Medicine*, 24(6), 569-573.

Kudchadkar, S. R., Aljohani, O. A., & Punjabi, N. M. (2014). Sleep of critically ill children in the pediatric intensive care unit: a systematic review. *Sleep Medicine Reviews*, 18(2), 103-110.

LaRosa, K. N., Crabtree, V. M., Jurbergs, N., & Harman, J. (2021). Behavioral sleep intervention to reduce bedsharing prior to stem cell transplant. *Journal of Clinical Sleep Medicine*, 17(2), 333-335.

McCarthy, M. C., Bastiani, J., & Williams, L. K. (2016). Are parenting behaviors associated with child sleep problems during treatment for acute lymphoblastic leukemia? *Cancer Medicine*, 5(7), 1473-1480.

McKenna, J. J., Ball, H. L., & Gettler, L. T. (2007). Mother–infant cosleeping, breastfeeding and sudden infant death syndrome: what biological anthropology has discovered about normal infant sleep and pediatric sleep medicine. *American Journal of Physical Anthropology: The Official Publication of the American Association of Physical Anthropologists*, 134(S45), 133-161.

McKenna, J. J., & Gettler, L. T. (2016). There is no such thing as infant sleep, there is no such thing as breastfeeding, there is only breastsleeping. *Acta Paediatrica*, 105(1), 17-21.

Monaghan, M., Herbert, L. J., Cogen, F. R., & Streisand, R. (2012). Sleep behaviors and parent functioning in young children with type 1 diabetes. *Children's Health*

Care, 41(3), 246-259.

Simon, A. K., Hollander, G. A., & McMichael, A. (2015). Evolution of the immune system in humans from infancy to old age. *Proceedings of the Royal Society B: Biological Sciences*, 282(1821), 20143085.

Thomaz, E. B. A. F., Cangussu, M. C. T., & Assis, A. M. O. (2012). Maternal breastfeeding, parafunctional oral habits and malocclusion in adolescents: a multivariate analysis. *International Journal of Pediatric Otorhinolaryngology*, 76(4), 500-506.

Urayama, K. Y., Buffler, P. A., Gallagher, E. R., Ayoob, J. M., & Ma, X. (2010). A meta-analysis of the association between day-care attendance and childhood acute lymphoblastic leukaemia. *International Journal of Epidemiology*, 39(3), 718-732.

Van Deuren, S., Boonstra, A., van Dulmen-den Broeder, E., Blijlevens, N., Knoop, H., & Loonen, J. (2020). Severe fatigue after treatment for childhood cancer. *Cochrane Database of Systematic Reviews*, (3).

Walter, L. M., Nixon, G. M., Davey, M. J., Downie, P. A., & Horne, R. S. (2015). Sleep and fatigue in pediatric oncology: A review of the literature. *Sleep Medicine Reviews*, 24, 71-82.

Zachek, C. M., Miller, M. D., Hsu, C., Schiffman, J. D., Sallan, S., Metayer, C., & Dahl, G. V. (2015). Children's cancer and environmental exposures: professional attitudes and practices. *Journal of Pediatric Hematology/Oncology*, 37(7), 491.

Zimmerman, D., Bartick, M., Feldman-Winter, L., Ball, H. L., & Academy of Breastfeeding Medicine. (2023). ABM Clinical Protocol# 37: Physiological Infant Care—Managing Nighttime Breastfeeding in Young Infants. *Breastfeeding Medicine*, 18(3), 159-168.

Chapter 8

Abela, K. M., Wardell, D., Rozmus, C., & LoBiondo-Wood, G. (2020). Impact of pediatric critical illness and injury on families: an updated systematic review. *Journal of Pediatric Nursing*, 51, 21-31.

Alderfer, M. A., Navsaria, N., & Kazak, A. E. (2009). Family functioning and posttraumatic stress disorder in adolescent survivors of childhood cancer. *Journal of Family Psychology*, 23(5), 717.

Bassi, G., Mancinelli, E., Di Riso, D., & Salcuni, S. (2021). Parental stress, anxiety and depression symptoms associated with self-efficacy in paediatric type 1 diabetes: a literature review. *International Journal of Environmental Research and Public Health*, 18(1), 152.

Bravo, L., Killela, M. K., Reyes, B. L., Santos, K. M. B., Torres, V., Huang, C. C., & Jacob, E. (2020). Self-management, self-efficacy, and health-related quality of life in children with chronic illness and medical complexity. *Journal of Pediatric Health Care*, 34(4), 304-314.

Büyüm, A. M., Kenney, C., Koris, A., Mkumba, L., & Raveendran, Y. (2020). Decolonising global health: if not now, when? *BMJ Global Health*, 5(8), e003394.

Chaput, J. P., Willumsen, J., Bull, F., Chou, R., Ekelund, U., Firth, J., ... & Katzmarzyk, P. T. (2020). 2020 WHO guidelines on physical activity and sedentary behaviour for children and adolescents aged 5–17 years: summary of the evidence. *International Journal of Behavioral Nutrition and Physical Activity*, 17, 1-9.

Cohen, S., Janicki-Deverts, D., Chen, E., & Matthews, K. A. (2010). Childhood socioeconomic status and adult health. *Annals of the New York Academy of Sciences*, 1186(1), 37-55.

Devonport, T. J., Ward, G., Morrissey, H., Burt, C., Harris, J., Burt, S., ... & Nicholls, W. (2023). A systematic review of inequalities in the mental health experiences of Black African, Black Caribbean and black-mixed UK populations: implications for action. *Journal of Racial and Ethnic Health Disparities*, 10(4), 1669-1681.

Dias, L. B., & Mendes-Castillo, A. M. C. (2021). The role of grandparents of children with cancer in the hospital. *Revista Brasileira de Enfermagem*, 74(5), e20201143-e20201143.

Eccleston, C., Wastell, S., Crombez, G., & Jordan, A. (2008). Adolescent social development and chronic pain. *European Journal of Pain*, 12(6), 765-774.

Flury, M., Orellana-Rios, C. L., Bergsträsser, E., & Becker, G. (2021). "This is the worst that has happened to me in 86 years": A qualitative study of the experiences of grandparents losing a grandchild due to a neurological or oncological disease. *Journal for Specialists in Pediatric Nursing*, 26(1), e12311.

Goosby, B. J. (2013). Early life course pathways of adult depression and chronic pain. *Journal of Health and Social Behavior*, 54(1), 75-91.

Haas, S. (2008). Trajectories of functional health: The 'long arm' of childhood health and socioeconomic factors. *Social Science & Medicine*, 66(4), 849-861.

Havill, N., Fleming, L. K., & Knafl, K. (2019). Well siblings of children with chronic illness: A synthesis research study. *Research in Nursing & Health*, 42(5), 334-348.

Houtepen, L. C., Heron, J., Suderman, M. J., Fraser, A., Chittleborough, C. R., & Howe, L. D. (2020). Associations of adverse childhood experiences with educational attainment and adolescent health and the role of family and socioeconomic factors: a prospective cohort study in the UK. *PLoS Medicine*, 17(3), e1003031.

Khandpur, N., Neri, D. A., Monteiro, C., Mazur, A., Frelut, M. L., Boyland, E., ... & Thivel, D. (2020). Ultra-processed food consumption among the paediatric population: an overview and call to action from the European childhood obesity group. *Annals of Nutrition and Metabolism*, 76(2), 109-113.

Long, K. A., Marsland, A. L., Wright, A., & Hinds, P. (2015). Creating a tenuous balance: Siblings' experience of a brother's or sister's childhood cancer diagnosis. *Journal of Pediatric Oncology Nursing*, 32(1), 21-31.

Lum, A., Wakefield, C. E., Donnan, B., Burns, M. A., Fardell, J. E., Jaffe, A., ... & Marshall, G. M. (2019). School students with chronic illness have unmet academic, social, and emotional school needs. *School Psychology*, 34(6), 627.

Kirkpatrick Johnson, M., Allen Berg, J., & Sirotzki, T. (2007). Differentiation in self-perceived adulthood: Extending the confluence model of subjective age identity. *Social Psychology Quarterly*, 70(3), 243-261.

Murray, C. B., Groenewald, C. B., de la Vega, R., & Palermo, T. M. (2020). Long-term impact of adolescent chronic pain on young adult educational, vocational, and social outcomes. *Pain*, 161(2), 439.

References

Novak-Pavlic, M., Abdel Malek, S., Rosenbaum, P., Macedo, L. G., & Di Rezze, B. (2022). A scoping review of the literature on grandparents of children with disabilities. *Disability and Rehabilitation*, 44(13), 3326-3348.

Nutbeam, D., & Lloyd, J. E. (2021). Understanding and responding to health literacy as a social determinant of health. *Annu Rev Public Health*, 42(1), 159-73.

Pinquart, M. (2014). Achievement of developmental milestones in emerging and young adults with and without pediatric chronic illness—a meta-analysis. *Journal of Pediatric Psychology*, 39(6), 577-587.

Prchal, A., & Landolt, M. A. (2012). How siblings of pediatric cancer patients experience the first time after diagnosis: a qualitative study. *Cancer Nursing*, 35(2), 133-140.

Qiu, Y., Xu, L., Pan, Y., He, C., Huang, Y., Xu, H., ... & Dong, C. (2021). Family resilience, parenting styles and psychosocial adjustment of children with chronic illness: a cross-sectional study. *Frontiers in Psychiatry*, 12, 646421.

Rosenberg, A. R., Bradford, M. C., Junkins, C. C., Taylor, M., Zhou, C., Sherr, N., ... & Joyce, P. (2019). Effect of the promoting resilience in stress management intervention for parents of children with cancer (PRISM-P): a randomized clinical trial. *JAMA Network Open*, 2(9), e1911578-e1911578.

Sadruddin, A. F., Ponguta, L. A., Zonderman, A. L., Wiley, K. S., Grimshaw, A., & Panter-Brick, C. (2019). How do grandparents influence child health and development? A systematic review. *Social Science & Medicine*, 239, 112476.

Settersten Jr, R. A., & Ray, B. (2010). What's going on with young people today? The long and twisting path to adulthood. *The Future of Children*, 19-41.

Shivers, C. M., Jackson, J. B., & McGregor, C. M. (2019). Functioning among typically developing siblings of individuals with autism spectrum disorder: A meta-analysis. *Clinical Child and Family Psychology Review*, 22, 172-196.

Tatterton, M. J., & Walshe, C. (2019). Understanding the bereavement experience of grandparents following the death of a grandchild from a life-limiting condition: A meta-ethnography. *Journal of Advanced Nursing*, 75(7), 1406-1417.

Van Schoors, M., De Mol, J., Laeremans, N., Verhofstadt, L. L., Goubert, L., & Van Parys, H. (2019). Siblings' experiences of everyday life in a family where one child is diagnosed with blood cancer: a qualitative study. *Journal of Pediatric Oncology Nursing*, 36(2), 131-142.

Verhoef, J. A., Miedema, H. S., Van Meeteren, J., Stam, H. J., & Roebroeck, M. E. (2013). A new intervention to improve work participation of young adults with physical disabilities: a feasibility study. *Developmental Medicine & Child Neurology*, 55(8), 722-728.

Winger, A., Kvarme, L. G., Løyland, B., Kristiansen, C., Helseth, S., & Ravn, I. H. (2020). Family experiences with palliative care for children at home: a systematic literature review. *BMC Palliative Care*, 19, 1-19.

Woodgate, R. L. (2006). Siblings' experiences with childhood cancer: a different way of being in the family. *Cancer Nursing*, 29(5), 406-414.

Yang, H. C., Mu, P. F., Sheng, C. C., Chen, Y. W., & Hung, G. Y. (2016). A systematic review of the experiences of siblings of children with cancer. *Cancer Nursing*, 39(3), E12-E21.

Index

A&E (Accident & Emergency) 30–2
acute illness 29–35, 121
acute on chronic illness 34–5
administrative hospital staff 45–6
adolescence 134
adult services, transition to 108
adverse childhood experiences (ACEs) 138–9, 146–7
advocacy 15, 111–12
age of child 74–5
Ainsworth, Margaret 67
allowances, making 42–3
anaesthesia 92–3, 94 *see also* general anaesthetic
anger 23, 42, 136, 152
antenatal diagnosis 22–3, 38–9
anxiety 25, 27–8, 42, 98
art therapists 53, 141
aspirations for children 19
asthma 9, 34, 82, 122
attachment 64–8, 77, 139
authoritative parenting 148
autism 138

Baby Friendly Standards 47–8
bags (for hospital), packing 62
bedsharing 125–8, 149
behaviour management 42–3
blood tests 49–50, 86–7
boredom in hospital 61–2
boundaries, keeping 42–3
Bowlby, John 65, 67
Brazelton, Thomas Berry 67
breastfeeding 56, 96, 102–3, 126
buccal medications 81
Butler, Roisin 40–1, 133–4, 152

cancer 15, 40, 122, 123, 136
cannulation 86–8
care plans 44, 132
catering in hospitals 46, 56–7 *see also* food

central lines 87, 105–6
cerebral palsy 122
chaplaincy 46
Chapman, Hannah 113–17
child-centred information 43
chronic conditions 18, 35–44, 121–4, 133–5
cleaning staff in hospitals 47, 60
clinical care in the home 99–107
clinical observations ('obs') 57–8, 69, 129
cognitive behavioural therapy 26
collaborative working models 69, 72–3, 106, 107–9 *see also* family-centred care
comfort objects 63, 128
community nursing teams 106
compassionate language 109–11, 150–1
complex needs 97–117
consent 80, 92–3
continence needs 106
continuity of care 108
coping mechanisms 15, 27–8
costs of hospital stays 70–1, 76, 99, 144, 149
CPAP (continuous positive airway pressure) masks 100, 101
creams/gels/ointments 83
critical care, family-centred 76 *see also* PICU (Paediatric Intensive Care Unit)
cry-it-out sleep training 123
CT scans 90
'cuddle hold' 88
cultural and religious needs 72, 75, 146, 151

death 112–17, 138, 142
debriefing 34
dental care 108
developmental checks 108

170

Index

developmental milestones 134–5
diabetes 9, 35, 39, 93, 122
diagnosis
    after birth 39–41
    antenatal diagnosis 22–3, 38–9
    psychological journey of 26–7
    role of paediatrician 49
dieticians 53, 102, 103
digital records 108
disappointment 17–19, 23
discharge 108, 131–2
dissociation 27
distraction techniques 28, 50, 88, 96
doctors 48–9, 55–6, 79–80
drug charts 59

ear medications 83
earaches 120
earplugs 62
ECGs 90
eczema 83–4, 122
education in hospital 52–3
effect on parents 13–28 *see also* supporting families
EMDR (eye movement desensitization and reprocessing) 26
Emerson, P. E. 65
emotional support for parents 12–16, 109, 152 *see also* supporting families
empathy 16, 17
end-of-life care 113
enteral feeding 103–4
epilepsy 9, 122, 135
equipment 107, 108
examinations 79–80
exercise 147–8
expectations of parents in terms of child's care 69
experts, parents become 43, 72, 98, 109, 112, 132
eye medicine 83

faith support 46
faltering growth 37
family integrated care (FIC) 77
family-centred approaches to sleep 129–31
family-centred care 64–78, 148–52
fasting 93–4
'feed and wrap' technique 90
feeding support at home 102–6
fighting for your children 15
finances 70–1, 76, 99, 144, 149
flare-ups of chronic illness 34–5, 42
food
    catering in hospitals 46, 56–7
    dieticians 53
    feeding support at home 102–6
    mealtimes in hospitals 56–7
    optimising diet 147
    parent kitchens 149
    for parents 56–7, 70–1, 150
    snacks 63
formula feeding 103
freeze response 20–2
Freud, Sigmund 66

gastroenteritis 120
general anaesthetic 89, 90
grab bags 62, 63
grandparents 141–3
gratitude 16, 21
Grey, Davina 142
grief 17–19, 110, 113–17, 142
guilt 18

Harlow, Harry 67
health inequalities 146–7
health records 71–2
healthcare assistants (HCAs) 47
healthcare workers
    effects on 16
    in hospitals 45–54
    pragmatism 18–19

high-dependency units 31 *see also* PICU (Paediatric Intensive Care Unit)
home comforts, bringing 61
home-based care 98–107
hope 15, 21, 99
hospices 108, 114–15
hospital stays *see also* PICU (Paediatric Intensive Care Unit)
   being with your child on the ward 34, 45–63
   family-centred care 64–78, 148–52
   food 46, 56–7, 70–1, 149
   improving hospital care 148–52
   parent beds 74, 76–7, 125, 149
   people who work in hospitals 45–54
   routines 54–61
   sleep 125–8
   staff 45–54
   treatments and procedures 79–96
   ward rounds 49, 55–6
   what to bring 62–3
housekeeping staff in hospitals 47, 60
housework 144

imaging scans 51
immunocompromised children 33, 41, 147
infant feeding 37–8, 47–8, 102
information-sharing in family-centred care 71–2, 107–9, 150–1
inhaled medications 82
injections 82–3
institutionalisation 18–19
intensive paediatric care 31, 40–1, 76, 108, 122, 137, 140
internet searching 28
interpreters 56, 72
intravenous medication/fluid 87–8
intravenous nutrition 105–6
intubation 41, 94 *see also* tube feeding

isolation (hospital isolation rooms) 28, 31, 62, 64
isolation (social isolation of parent and/or child) 70, 98, 145

joined-up care 12, 107–9

language barriers 56
laundry 62, 71, 74, 144
leukaemia 40–1, 112, 123
life-limiting diagnoses 112–17
lifts/logistical help for families 145
lights in hospitals 60–1
listening to parents 42
litigation, fear of 91
loneliness 70, 76, 145
long-term impacts on children 133–5
long-term ventilation (LTV) 101
love 21, 99
lumbar punctures 89

Maillardet, Hannah 22–3
mealtimes 56–7
medical opinion, when to seek 32–3
medication
   daily routines in hospital 58–9
   helping children take 84–6
   long-term 42
   pain relief 96
   role of pharmacists 49
   and sleep 128
   treatments 81–6
mental health impacts *see also* anxiety; psychological support; stress
   benefits of family-centred care 69
   on families 26, 71, 99, 109–11, 137, 138
   numbness 20–2, 25
   pre-existing conditions exacerbated 131
   on siblings 138

Index

on sick children 133–5
mental load 109
minimisation 18–19
mouth-breathing 120, 122–3
MRI scans 90
music therapists 53, 141

names, using 75
nappies 106
nasal medication 82
nasogastric tubes 104–5
nebulisers 82
negotiation in family-centred care 73
Neonatal Intensive Care 21
neonatal nursing 37–8
'new normal' 23–4
Nixon, Gemma 25–6, 148–50
noise in hospitals 60–1, 131
non-pharmacological pain relief 96
normality, disruption to 23–5
'not what was planned' 22–4
numbing cream 86, 88
numbness 20–2, 25
nursery nurses 47
nurses 48, 52, 55, 58
nursing, expecting parents to undertake 69

'obs' (clinical observations) 57–8, 69, 129
occupational therapy 53, 107
ocular medications 83
optimising wellness 146–8
optimism 15
oral feeding 102
oral medications 81
otic medication 83
over-identification 17
over-protection 25
oxygen support 100–1

packing a bag 62
paediatric A&E 30–1

paediatric nurses 48
paediatricians 48–9, 55–6, 80
pain 58, 95–6
pain relief 96
pain scores 58, 96
palliative care 112–17, 138–9
parasympathetic nervous system 124
parenteral nutrition 49, 53, 105–6
partnerships with parents 69, 72–3, 106, 107–9 *see also* family-centred care
paying it forward 151–2
PEG (percutaneous endoscopic gastrostomy) tube 105
people who work in hospitals 45–54
person-first language 75
pets 144
PEW (paediatric early warning) score 57–8
pharmacists 49, 108
pharmacological pain relief 96
phlebotomists 49–50
physiotherapy 54
Piaget, Jean 66
PICU (Paediatric Intensive Care Unit) 31, 40–1, 76, 108, 122, 137, 140
Piper, Brittney 95, 139, 148–9
Platt Report 67, 68
play specialists 50, 53, 61–2, 88, 90
play therapy 50, 139, 141
play/childhood activities 43–4, 50
PMTS (paediatric medical traumatic stress) 99
porters 50–1
positive language 109–11
practical help for families 143–4
pregnancy, diagnosis during 22–3, 38–9
prematurity 35–8, 100
pre-op assessments 92–3
Prescott, James 68
pressure sores 106

privacy/dignity 9, 22, 60, 74, 76, 80, 134
procedures 86–92 *see also* examinations; tests
protecting children 43–4
proximity-seeking behaviours 66
psychological maturity 135
psychological support
    for parents 25–6, 108, 109
    for siblings 138, 141
psychological therapies 42, 50, 51
psychotherapists 51
PTSD (post-traumatic stress disorder) 25–6, 98–9, 136
'putting a brave face on it' 18–19

radiologists and radiographers 51
rapid deterioration 33–4
rectal medications 81
'red book' 71–2
relapse and remission 35
relationship strain (parents) 70, 99
religious needs 72, 75
research/learning about child's condition 39 *see also* experts, parents become
resilience 15, 23, 99, 139, 148
respiratory support (at home) 100–1
respite 108, 145
resuscitation 91
risk assessment 130
Rosales, Shurron 27, 109–11
routines in hospitals 45–54, 128
Rutter, Michael 68
Rycroft, Matthew 152

safeguarding 52
scans 89–90
Schaeffer, H. R. 65
school in hospital 52–3
Schore, Allan 68
sedation 122
self-care 34

self-limiting illnesses 32–3
sensory overload 60–1
separation anxiety 67
serious, rapid illness 33–4
shift changes 55
shock 39, 40
siblings 53, 70, 108, 135–41
side-car cribs 126–7
SIDS (Sudden Infant Death Syndrome) 126
signposting to support 110–11
skin care at home 106–7
skin medication 83–4
skin-to-skin 96
sleep 118–32
    bedsharing 125–8, 149
    oxygen support 101
    parent beds 74, 76–7, 125, 149
    PICU 76
sleep apnoea 101
sleep pathology 101, 122–3
sleep recovery after hospital admission 131–2
sleep training 123
Smith, Amanda 37–8
smoothies/juices 34
social histories 136
social media 139, 152
social model of disability 111
social workers 51–2, 99
solid food 103
specialist nurses 48, 107
speech and language therapy 54, 102, 103
spinning plates 9–10, 71
Spitz, Rene 67
staff, hospital 45–54
stoma bags 106
strengths-based approaches 152
strengths-based language 151
stress
    age of child 24–5
    automatic stress responses 27–8

Index

caring for sick children at home 98, 99
disruption to family life 18, 24
and long-term outcomes 147
optimising wellness 148
parent stressors 70–1, 109
and sleep 124
stress-informed practice 131
treatments and procedures 91–2
student healthcare workers 52, 91
support groups 39
supporting children with chronic illness 43–4
supporting families 133–52 *see also* family-centred care
  chronic conditions 42–4
  emotional support for parents 12–16, 109, 152
  ensuring nutrition and breaks 34
  grandparents 141–3
  how to support families of sick children 143–6
  parents accompanying a child in hospital 61, 74
  psychological support 25–6, 108, 109, 138, 141
  siblings 135–41
  therapy (for children) 50, 53–4
  therapy (for parents) 26
supporting staff/colleagues 34 *see also* family-centred care
surgery 92–6
sympathetic nervous system 124

talking therapies 42, 51, 141
Taylor, Michelle 43–4
teachers in hospitals 52–3
terminal illness 112–17
tests 31, 79–80, 86–91
therapy (for children) 50, 53–4
therapy (for parents) 26
thief, childhood illness as a 14
thriving through illness 14, 134
tissue viability nurses 106
TPN (total parenteral nutrition) 49, 53, 105–6
tracheostomy tubes 101
trainees/students 52, 91
training for parents 108
transdermal medication 84
transfer planning 108
transport 108
trauma (parental) 20, 25–6, 76, 98, 131
trauma-informed practice 131
triage 31
tube feeding 53, 103–5
tube medications 81

ultrasound scans 89–90
underlying conditions, children with 33
upper respiratory tract infections (URTIs) 120

vigilance, constant 42
visitors 62, 145

wards *see* hospital stays
Watson, John 66
Watson, Shelley 136–8
weekends in hospital 59
wellness, optimising 146–8
'why me/my child' 42
work/employment 71, 137, 145

X-rays 90–1

Young, Catherine 20–1

Available from Pinter & Martin
in the Why it Matters series

1. *Why Your Baby's Sleep Matters* Sarah Ockwell-Smith
2. *Why Hypnobirthing Matters* Katrina Berry
3. *Why Doulas Matter* Maddie McMahon
4. *Why Postnatal Depression Matters* Mia Scotland
5. *Why Babywearing Matters* Rosie Knowles
6. *Why the Politics of Breastfeeding Matter* Gabrielle Palmer
7. *Why Breastfeeding Matters* Charlotte Young
8. *Why Starting Solids Matters* Amy Brown
9. *Why Human Rights in Childbirth Matter* Rebecca Schiller
10. *Why Mothers' Medication Matters* Wendy Jones
11. *Why Home Birth Matters* Natalie Meddings
12. *Why Caesarean Matters* Clare Goggin
13. *Why Mothering Matters* Maddie McMahon
14. *Why Induction Matters* Rachel Reed
15. *Why Birth Trauma Matters* Emma Svanberg
16. *Why Oxytocin Matters* Kerstin Uvnäs Moberg
17. *Why Breastfeeding Grief and Trauma Matter* Amy Brown
18. *Why Postnatal Recovery Matters* Sophie Messager
19. *Why Pregnancy and Postnatal Exercise Matter* Rehana Jawadwala
20. *Why Baby Loss Matters* Kay King
21. *Why Infant Reflux Matters* Carol Smyth
22. *Why Tongue-tie Matters* Sarah Oakley
23. *Why Formula Feeding Matters* Shel Banks
24. *Why Grandmothers Matter* Naomi Stadlen
25. *Why Mixed Feeding Matters* Karen Hall
26. *Why Single Parents Matter* Amy Brown
27. *Why Childhood Illness Matters* Lyndsey Hookway

Series editor: Susan Last

pinterandmartin.com